Natural
approaches to
DIABETES

D1412364

Dr Sarah Brewer

piatkus

PIATKUS

First published in Great Britain in 2005 by Piatkus Books
This paperback edition published in 2010 by Piatkus

A CIP catalogue record for this book
is available from the British Library

ISBN 978-0-7499-4195-6

Typeset by Palimpsest Book Production, Grangemouth, Stirlingshire
Printed and bound in Great Britain by
CPI Mackays, Chatham ME5

Papers used by Piatkus are natural, renewable and recyclable
products sourced from well-managed forests and certified
in accordance with the rules of the Forest Stewardship Council.

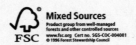

Mixed Sources
Product group from well-managed
forests and other controlled sources
www.fsc.org Cert no. SGS-COC-004081
© 1996 Forest Stewardship Council
FSC

Piatkus
An imprint of
Little, Brown Book Group
100 Victoria Embankment
London EC4Y 0DY

An Hachette UK Company
www.hachette.co.uk

www.piatkus.co.uk

Contents

Acknowledgements   iv

Introduction   v

1   Diabetes and metabolic syndrome: The basics   1

2   Long-term complications   21

3   Medical management   41

4   Lowering your risk   51

5   Healthy eating: The basics   67

6   Losing weight   92

7   Nutritional supplements: The basics   106

8   Antioxidants   123

9   The B vitamins   150

10   Minerals   174

11   Herbal medicines   195

12   Essential fatty acids   223

13   Putting it all together   235

Appendix 1   241

Appendix 2   245

Appendix 3   249

Notes   255

Bibliography   286

Index   287

Acknowledgements

Thanks to everyone who has helped with this book – it turned into a real labour of love! In particular I would like to thank Barbara Kiser who has helped to make sense of the wealth of clinical and research information, and make it more accessible. I would also like to thank those lecturing within the MSC course on Nutritional Medicine at the University of Surrey – their efforts are vital to help raise awareness of just how much research is available on nutritional approaches to wellness and disease.

Introduction

As you have picked up this book, it's more than likely that diabetes has touched your life in some way. You or someone close to you may have just been diagnosed and you could be feeling apprehensive or frightened at this sudden shift from 'well' to 'ill'. Your mind may be teeming with questions – why you have it, whether you can still eat your favourite foods, possible cures – and you may suddenly find yourself trawling bookshops and the Web, only to become bewildered by the vast array of information on offer.

On the other hand, you may have had the disease for some time, and simply be wondering whether the treatment you're following is the best for you. In either case, you want to know more.

And that is what you'll find here: this book is the only one you need to tell you all about the condition and the best treatments for it. As a former GP and seasoned health professional, I give you the most recent and reliable medical research on both types 1 and 2 diabetes, as well as the 'pre-diabetic' condition known as metabolic syndrome.

The bulk of this book, however, focuses on new ways of treating the condition, with the emphasis on natural methods such as diet, lifestyle, supplements and herbal medicines.

The fact that you can manage diabetes holistically is a relatively recent discovery. Not so long ago, insulin injections and pills were thought to be the only way to control the condition. But by the 1990s it had become increasingly clear that eating well, exercising and using the right herbs and micronutrients can reduce the need for drugs and injections in many people with type 2 diabetes, and prevent the condition in 'pre-diabetics'. For people with type 1 diabetes, natural treatments can work in tandem with injections to prevent the serious complications that can result from this potentially debilitating and sometimes deadly disease.

The close link between diet and exercise and type 2 diabetes is clearly shown by the fact that overweight and obesity are major factors in developing the condition. Obese women, for instance, are a staggering 27 times more likely to develop diabetes than women of normal weight. And it is the rising tide of overweight and obesity that is fuelling a worldwide epidemic of the disease.

Some 1.4 million people in the UK have been diagnosed with diabetes, while another million are believed to remain undiagnosed. The figure in the US is much higher, amounting to over 6 per cent of the population. Worldwide, the World Health Organization estimates that 150 million people have diabetes, and predicts that numbers may double by the year 2025.

It's clear, then, that there is an urgent need for an approach to diabetes that really works and is relatively free of harmful side effects. Fortunately, the natural, holistic options I present in this book offer just that. Living and eating well, and losing weight if you need to, are the basics. Then there is the wealth of vitamins, minerals, antioxidants and herbal remedies that are emerging as effective treatments for the condition. If any of that sounds daunting, rest assured that a sensible eating plan is easy to source and put together, as well as delicious and a breeze to follow – while the supplements and remedies are widely available.

Often, popular health books contain a number of case histories showing how making certain changes to diet and lifestyle has helped certain individuals. Although anecdotal evidence can be reassuring for many people, I have decided against including personal stories here. My book contains over 400 published references, the majority of which are published in peer-reviewed journals; many are randomised controlled trials – the gold standard evidence for assessing the benefits of different approaches. I hope this provides the reassurance that you and your healthcarers might need when considering whether or not to take certain supplements or to reduce your carbohydrate intake. Also, everyone is different, and this is especially true for people with diabetes – what suits one individual may not help another. That's why it is so important to monitor your glucose levels carefully when making any changes to your normal dietary, exercise and supplement routine.

The natural way with diabetes

The conventional approach to controlling diabetes has focused mainly on macronutrients – that is, carbohydrates, fats and proteins. But micronutrients – vitamins, minerals and antioxidants – are essential for health, and some can lower glucose and insulin levels as well as reduce the development of complications in people with both types 1 and 2 diabetes. Sadly, their advantages are not often discussed, as many doctors and dieticians wrongly believe you can get all the vitamins and minerals you need from your food.

We now know that this often isn't true. Vitamins can be destroyed by poor food processing, storage and preparation methods, and on top of that, people with diabetes may have a greater need for certain nutrients, making deficiencies more likely. In fact, the evidence suggests that lack of some vitamins and minerals may affect your blood glucose control and increase your risk of developing diabetes in the first place. In any case, many people are failing to get even the recommended daily amount of many micronutrients, and the number of people deficient in vitamins and minerals – as shown by the British government's own National Diet and Nutrition Survey – makes sobering reading (see page 109). All this strengthens the case immeasurably for taking the right nutritional supplements.

An interesting article[1] in the journal *Medical Hypotheses*, for instance, suggests that it may now be feasible to target each of the main abnormalities associated with type 2 diabetes using specific nutritional supplements. The paper suggests that the mineral chromium and conjugated linoleic acid – a fatty acid found in meat and dairy products – can help body cells overcome insulin resistance (see page 232); that the B vitamin biotin may help lower production of new blood sugar in the liver; and that the antioxidant co-enzyme Q10 may improve the working of the insulin-producing cells in the pancreas.

Even single supplements can have a profound effect. In one study, a group of healthy men aged 42 to 60 took above-average amounts of vitamin E for four years. Compared to this group, a control group who supplemented with below-average amounts were found to be nearly four times more likely to develop type 2 diabetes at the end of the test period. But that is only one of the startling findings revealed later in this book.

Another important strand in treating diabetes naturally is herbal medicine. Over 400 traditional plant treatments for diabetes have been recorded, yet most have yet to be evaluated. In 2003,[2] a review of the evidence for the effectiveness and safety of herbal, vitamin and mineral therapies in people with diabetes looked at 108 clinical trials involving 4565 people with diabetes or impaired glucose tolerance. Among these studies were 58 controlled clinical trials of certain herbal treatments. The evidence for an improvement in control of blood sugar was positive in over three-quarters of these trials – and very few adverse effects were reported.

Thankfully, a growing number of people are getting the message, as was shown in a survey of 500 people with diabetes. This found that 44 per cent were taking over-the-counter supplements, and 31 per cent were using alternative medicines. As the authors wrote: 'The money spent on alternative and non-prescription supplements nearly equals that spent on prescription medications. In view of the money spent in this area the time is past due to evaluate these remedies and to establish what merit they have.'[3]

I wholeheartedly agree with them, and in this book I show the research behind some of the supplements that may prove helpful for people with diabetes. A great deal of it is new, and heralds inspiring developments in treating the disease. But this is not the moment to plunge into a brand-new regime regardless. If you choose to take any supplements, it is very important that you read the following warning.

WARNING

Complementary approaches should always support the medical treatment your doctor has recommended, and should never take the place of normal medical care. Never stop taking any prescribed medications except under the advice of your doctor. Only take supplements with the full permission of your doctor.

Always monitor blood glucose levels carefully when starting to take a supplement and discuss any changes in your glucose control with your GP. You must make sure you know what you should do if your glucose control changes in any way.

Only use supplements – especially herbal remedies – under the supervision of a medical herbalist or doctor if you are already taking drugs to lower blood glucose levels. This is very important to prevent hypoglycaemic attacks.

Note especially: This book is not intended for women who are pregnant or who develop gestational diabetes.

How to use this book

If you have only recently been diagnosed, or feel your knowledge about diabetes needs updating, I would suggest reading the first chapters first, to discover what you can about the condition. Chapter 1 tells you all you need to know about the causes and symptoms of diabetes and metabolic syndrome. Chapter 2 looks at the long-term complications that can develop if your glucose control is not kept as tight as it should be, while Chapter 3 goes through the day-to-day medical management of diabetes, such as insulin injections. Chapter 4 examines ways of lowering your risk of developing type 2 diabetes and metabolic syndrome.

You can, however, skip to diets or supplements directly if you wish. If you just want to know about general rules for healthy eating, jump to Chapter 5. Weight-loss diets – stressing the benefits of the low-carbohydrate approach – are covered in Chapter 6, as overweight and obesity are major risk factors for developing type 2 diabetes. The rest of the book looks at what nutritional supplements – antioxidants, vitamins, minerals, herbal medicines and essential fatty acids – have to offer.

If you're new to supplements, rest assured that they are widely available in chemists, supermarkets and healthfood stores. For those preferring to use mail order, I can recommend The Nutri Centre (tel: 020 7323 2382; www.nutricentre.com) and Healthspan (tel: 0800 73 123 77; www.healthspan.co.uk).

The chapters on nutritional medicine are fully referenced to so you can investigate further if you wish. Further information on some of the key research, which I feel is exceptionally important, is also available in the appendices of this book.

Diabetes and metabolic syndrome: The basics

Developing a detailed understanding of diabetes or the pre-diabetic condition metabolic syndrome might look a challenging task, particularly if you've just been diagnosed. You may be feeling especially vulnerable, and as if the last thing you need is to 'have your nose rubbed in it'. But what you may find instead is that knowing all you can about diabetes will make it seem far less intimidating – and will give you the grounding you need to make informed choices about healthy eating plans and supplements. Remember, though, that while the focus of this book is on natural approaches, these are meant to *complement* your doctor's treatment, not replace it.

What is diabetes?

Diabetes mellitus is a chronic disorder described in the oldest known medical document in the world – the 3500-year-old Ebers papyrus from Egypt – so the condition has been with us for at least that long, and probably longer.

In essence, diabetes happens when levels of glucose in your bloodstream are consistently too high. But to understand the condition fully, we need to untangle the workings of glucose and the other main player in this drama, the hormone insulin.

Insulin is produced by the pancreas, a gland that nestles behind the duodenum; but we mainly obtain glucose, which is one of the body's primary fuels, from the carbohydrates we eat. When grains

1

and other carbohydrates are digested, they enter the bloodstream as glucose. The blood sugar is then 'escorted' by insulin into muscle and fat cells, which use it for energy, while excess glucose is stored as the starchy substance glycogen, or as fat. The following box gives a detailed picture of this fascinating choreography.

Insulin and glucose: a matter of balance

To understand diabetes, it's vital to see how insulin and glucose work together.

Insulin is made in so-called beta cells in the pancreas, found within clusters of specialised cells known as the islets of Langerhans. Normally, about a million of these islets are scattered among the other pancreatic cells, which make digestive juices.

Glucose – which is what our cells use for fuel – is obtained when carbohydrate foods, such as potatoes, bread, pasta, rice, sugar and the like, are broken down in the process of digestion. Starchy or sugary foods such as bread, for instance, break down directly into glucose, while fruit contains the simple sugar fructose, which is converted during digestion into glucose. As the glucose travels down your gut it is absorbed into your bloodstream, first passing through your liver, where much of it is stored.

When your beta cells detect a raised level of glucose (after you've eaten a sandwich or a baked potato, for instance), they release a quick pulse of insulin over a few minutes. As a result, insulin levels suddenly peak, then fall. This is followed by a second, more sustained release of insulin which continues for an hour or more before dropping back to a low level of output. Insulin is therefore secreted at low levels between meals and at an increased level during mealtimes.

Once secreted, insulin escorts glucose out of the bloodstream and into your muscle and fat cells. The hormone manages this vital task by encouraging specially shaped receptors to move from inside the cell to the cell walls, where they allow glucose to enter, as if through a door. Once in, glucose is either burnt for energy, or is stored in the liver and muscles as glycogen, which acts as an emergency fuel source. The body can then use glycogen when levels of glucose in the blood fall – for instance, when you're exercising hard at the gym.

So insulin is, in essence, the key regulator of our blood sugar levels. Aside from helping to ferry glucose into cells, insulin can also have a balancing effect by suppressing or switching off the production of new glucose within the liver from stored glycogen (see page 17). At any one time, your blood glucose levels depend on the amount of glucose you absorb from your intestines during mealtimes, plus the amount of glucose made and released in your liver, minus the amount taken up by your body cells.

This task of insulin and glucose – keeping the body's engine running – is finely tuned. Diabetes throws a spanner in the works, however, by disrupting the production and release of insulin.

There are different reasons for this critical upset, corresponding to the different types of diabetes (see below). The pancreas may stop making insulin altogether, may no longer make enough to meet the body's needs, or may produce so much that your cells fail to respond to it – a condition known as insulin resistance (see page 4). The end result of all of these scenarios is that too much glucose remains in the bloodstream.

Normally, your blood glucose levels are maintained within quite narrow limits (just under 4 to 8 millimoles per litre, expressed as 4mmol/l to 8mmol/l) and average out at around 5mmol/l. But if you have diabetes, glucose will quickly build up in your bloodstream, partly because the fat and muscle cells cannot absorb it, and partly because your liver keeps pushing new glucose into the circulation. Diabetes is diagnosed when your blood glucose levels rise above normal levels.

Types of diabetes

Types 1 and 2

There are two main types of diabetes mellitus: type 1 and type 2.

If you have type 1 diabetes, you will most likely have developed it when relatively young, and be relatively slim. Type 1 tends to affect children and young people, and be diagnosed between the ages of 10 and 15 – although it can strike at any time. It is a lifelong, severe chronic disease, and the most common one of childhood.

Type 1 develops when a person has a very low level of insulin; thus it has been known as 'insulin-dependent' diabetes, as people with the condition must rely on regular injections of the hormone. It is thought to be an autoimmune condition, meaning that your immune system attacks something within your own body – in this case, most, or all, of the beta cells in your pancreas. Type 1 diabetes accounts for just a fifth of the cases in Europe and North America.

Type 2 diabetes in these regions is much more common, making up the remaining 80 per cent. Once called non-insulin dependent or maturity-onset diabetes, type 2 tends to occur in people over 30. Four out of five people with this kind of diabetes are very overweight, and for men and women both, the risk of developing the condition increases as their weight goes up. Not everyone with type 2 is overweight, however, so people with it are classified as having either obese or non-obese type 2 diabetes.

You can still produce insulin if you have type 2, but it will either not be enough to control your blood glucose levels, or, paradoxically, be so much that the body becomes unable to respond to it properly. The latter condition, known as insulin resistance, is very common in overweight or obese people.

Insulin resistance

Overweight and insulin resistance often go hand in hand, and both can be characteristics of type 2 diabetes or the pre-diabetic condition metabolic syndrome (see page 16). In essence, someone who is overweight or obese is likely to be eating a lot of simple carbohydrates – white bread, sugary cakes and biscuits, sweets and so on. Every time they have a carbohydrate 'hit', their beta cells will release a burst of insulin. So if they're snacking on this kind of food many times a day, tissue cells will start to become desensitised to the flood of insulin, and fail to respond to it properly. In other words, they become insulin resistant.

When this happens, the normally rapid response to glucose in the bloodstream is reduced, so blood glucose levels remain higher than normal, for longer than normal, after eating a meal. Over time, pre-diabetic conditions or type 2 diabetes can develop. (See page 17 for a more detailed discussion of insulin resistance.)

There can be other problems in type 2 diabetes. The insulin you produce may not be packaged as well as normal, so that more insulin building blocks and incomplete chains of insulin are released from beta cells, instead of the normal, active insulin.

Other forms of diabetes

There are rarer forms of diabetes. Sometimes, diabetes is classified by a pre-existing medical condition. For instance, if you have pancreatic disease or hormone problems – whether caused by medications, abnormalities of insulin or its receptors, or genetic syndromes – your diabetes may be classified according to that underlying cause.

Taking corticosteroids, which mimic hormones produced by the adrenal glands, or thiazide diuretics can nudge you towards diabetes. But more common is the form of diabetes that develops in some women during pregnancy.

Diabetes during pregnancy

Known as gestational diabetes, this type occurs when the pancreas does not make enough insulin to cope with the extra demands pregnancy imposes on the body. It is relatively rare, affecting around 5 per cent of non-diabetic women (between 1 and 2 per cent of women who become pregnant already have diabetes). In true gestational diabetes, blood sugar levels usually return to normal soon after the baby is delivered.

But some women aren't so fortunate. As gestational diabetes is a sign that the pancreas cannot cope with extra strain, three out of four women who develop it go on to develop type 2 diabetes in later life. Taking preventative measures, however, can go some way towards staving it off or diminishing this risk considerably.

Signs and symptoms

How would you know whether you have diabetes? Some people – and you might have been one – have no symptoms at all, and their diabetes is picked up during a routine check-up at their clinic. But the symptoms of diabetes, if you have them, are quite distinct. If you experience any of them, it's vital that you go to your doctor for an immediate test.

Type 1 symptoms

Because type 1 diabetes so frequently strikes children, parents would do well to become familiar with the symptoms.

Excessive urination The word diabetes actually means 'excessive urination', and one of the main symptoms of untreated type 1 diabetes is producing more urine than normal – a condition known as polyuria. So if you find yourself going to the toilet far more than you usually do, yet haven't been drinking more water than usual, take this symptom seriously.

Polyuria happens with type 1 diabetes because the excess glucose in your system overspills through your kidneys, and pulls water with it due to the process of osmosis. As a result, you can produce five times as much urine as you normally do, and need to use the toilet in the night-time as well as the day. In the process, you may also lose water-soluble vitamins and minerals, which is one of the reasons micronutrient levels are often depleted in people with diabetes. Someone with untreated diabetes can lose as much as

1kg sugar through their urine per day – equivalent to 4000kcal – so they can also experience rapid weight loss (see below).

Thirst Because people with type 1 are losing so much fluid, they can become very thirsty, and even experience a dry mouth despite drinking litres of water. If you find yourself quaffing far more water than you usually do with little effect on your thirst, be wary.

Weight loss and exhaustion Often, people with type 1 diabetes are much hungrier and eat more, yet lose weight rapidly. As we've seen, this is mainly down to polyuria. Glucose cannot enter body cells and it builds up in the circulation until it reaches a level at which it overspills into the urine. You are therefore urinating away one of your body's main fuel sources, so it's not surprising that tiredness, listlessness and fatigue are major symptoms. Meanwhile, the extra sugar in your circulation can encourage infections such as cystitis, thrush and boils.

Blurred vision Some people with undiagnosed diabetes also complain of blurred vision. This happens because excess glucose in the blood alters the consistency of body fluids, and the eye lens can actually swell. This produces a temporary short-sightedness which disappears once sugar levels are back under normal control.

If you are having these symptoms, don't delay your trip to the doctor. Type 1 diabetes will eventually lead to a diabetic coma if it remains undiagnosed and untreated. This is triggered by a build-up of chemicals and acids in the blood, a condition known as ketoacidosis, which happens when starving cells, which cannot obtain glucose from your circulation, develop a very abnormal metabolism. Diabetic coma is a medical emergency, and it will need immediate treatment in intensive care.

Type 2 symptoms

The symptoms of uncontrolled type 2 diabetes are more or less the same as those for type 1, but they tend to develop more slowly and are usually less severe. So if you have type 2 diabetes, it may well have been picked up during a routine medical examination rather than through your having reported any specific health complaints.

Type 2 symptoms are also less specific and can include a lack of energy, listlessness and general weariness. Obesity is also common. As with type 1 diabetes, you may have been having recurrent infections – the result of high glucose levels in the blood – and this is often how the condition is first suspected and diagnosed.

On average, there is a delay of between 9 and 12 years before someone with type 2 diabetes is diagnosed. This is unacceptable, so if you suspect you might have symptoms of diabetes, ask to be screened without delay.

What causes diabetes?

As we've seen, diabetes happens when the pancreas fails to produce enough insulin to meet your body's needs. In most people with type 1 diabetes, the destruction of beta cells by the body's own immune system sets the stage for this condition. We still don't know what triggers this immune reaction.

Type 2 diabetes usually results from insulin resistance (see page 4), one of the features of which is abnormal insulin secretion. Again, it's poorly understood why this happens. The most popular theory is that inheriting certain genes predisposes you towards developing diabetes, but that another trigger is needed to cause the condition itself. This trigger may be a viral illness that damages the insulin-secreting beta cells in some way, or that sets off the production of abnormal antibodies that attack and destroy beta cells.

Whatever the cause, let's take a look at the latest research on what triggers both type 1 and type 2 diabetes.

Heredity

Diabetes tends to run in families, and that suggests that certain genes are involved. Not everybody who inherits these genes will develop diabetes, however. Overall, the chance of a baby with one diabetic parent developing diabetes at some point throughout life is around 1 in 100. However, the child has a greater chance of developing diabetes – between 1 in 20 and 1 in 40 – if their father is diabetic; if only their mother is, their chances are between 1 in 40 and 1 in 80. If both parents are diabetic, the chance of the child developing diabetes at some stage in their life is around 1 in 20.

A number of genes have been found to be linked with diabetes. With type 1, the strongest link is a gene called HLA-DR, which is involved in starting immune responses, including one that might attack beta cells. In type 2 diabetes, a number of genes that control insulin secretion and action have also been identified.

Among young identical twins, if one develops type 1 diabetes, there is only a 30 to 50 per cent chance that the other twin will develop it as well, even though they share identical genes. The link is much higher for type 2 diabetes: there is a 90 per cent chance that if one twin is affected, the other will also develop the disease.

The environment within the womb during a foetus's development may play a role in the risk of developing diabetes. For example, babies with the lowest birth weight appear to be more likely to develop type 2 diabetes in later life – possibly due to lack of certain nutrients in the womb which may affect the way beta cells learn to produce insulin, or the way muscle and fat cells learn to respond to insulin. Other health problems such as coronary heart disease, metabolic syndrome and high blood pressure have also been linked with low birth weight.

Ethnic background

The number of people with type 1 diabetes varies hugely between countries. This form of diabetes is very prevalent in Finland and Sweden, yet very low in Japan, China and Korea. In fact, someone living in Finland is 10 times more likely to develop type 1 diabetes compared with someone in Macedonia. Overall, type 1 diabetes is more common in Europeans, and type 2 more common in Hispanics and African-Americans. What all this tells us is that environmental or ethnic factors, as well as genetic material passed down within our families, may also influence whether or not someone develops diabetes.

Immune attack

In over 90 per cent of cases, type 1 diabetes is caused by the destruction of beta cells in the pancreas by the person's own immune system. And when examined under a microscope, the islets of Langerhans (see page 2) of people newly diagnosed with type 1 diabetes are very inflamed. In most of these people, anti-bodies aimed against parts of the body, such as beta cells, insulin or an enzyme produced mainly by islet cells and known as glutamic acid decarboxylase, or GAD, can usually be detected as well. These immune processes destroy insulin-producing cells so that people with established type 1 diabetes often have no beta cells left in their pancreas. In type 2 diabetes, however, there is no evidence of any involvement from the immune system. In this form of diabetes, around 50 per cent of the islet cells usually remain intact.

Build-up of amylin

If you have type 2 diabetes, the main abnormality visible under a microscope is a build-up of amylin – an insoluble, starch-like substance made from sugar and protein – around the islet cells. Amylin is produced in the beta cells and secreted together with insulin, but for some reason it can accumulate, and actually inhibit insulin secretion in some people. Why this happens, and the role it plays in causing type 2, is still the subject of intense study.

Drugs

I've mentioned above (page 5) how some forms of diabetes can be triggered by drugs. A number of prescription drugs are known to increase blood glucose levels, including corticosteroids and drugs used to treat high blood pressure. In particular, doctors were recently warned against prescribing a combination of two drugs used to treat high blood pressure – a thiazide diuretic and a beta blocker – because researchers analysing data from seven trials involving over 70,000 people have found that people taking them together are 20 per cent more likely to develop type 2 diabetes compared with those on other treatments. The two types of drug should now only be used together where the benefits are thought to outweigh the risks.

Cold weather

Interestingly, type 1 diabetes is more likely to be diagnosed during winter than summer. This might be because the need for insulin increases during cold weather (for example, to push more glucose into muscle cells, to generate heat via shivering), or may be linked to environmental factors such as exposure to winter infections, or to levels of vitamin D (see page 52).

Viral infections

Scientists have noted that infection with mumps, rubella (German measles) or Coxsackie B viruses (which cause diseases ranging from mild stomach complaints to heart damage) may be linked with the development of diabetes, but there is not yet enough evidence to prove any firm connections in humans. In mice and rats, however, at least one virus that attacks the heart and brain is also known to cause diabetes – often within three days of infection – because the virus likes to live and grow within the beta cells, which are then attacked and destroyed by the immune system.

Diet

There is some evidence to suggest that if women eat a lot of smoked meat at the time of conception, they are more likely to have a child who develops type 1 diabetes. This may be because of the presence of harmful chemicals, nitrosamines, in smoked foods. Early weaning onto cows' milk may also increase the risk of a child developing type 1, possibly because the body makes antibodies against albumin protein in the milk, which might then cross-react with, and attack, beta cells. Again, this isn't proven, however.

With type 2 diabetes, diet is much more clearly a trigger in susceptible people. If you eat a lot of carbohydrates – particularly refined, sugary foods such as white bread, cakes, biscuits and sweets – you are more likely to become overweight or obese, and develop the pre-diabetic condition metabolic syndrome, as well as type 2 diabetes.

We'll be learning about healthy diets for diabetes in Chapters 5 and 6, as well as in Appendix 3.

Toxins

Some toxins are known to trigger diabetes in animals, and the rat poison, vacor, can cause type 1 diabetes in humans. It is therefore possible that environmental toxins that have not yet been identified may be responsible for causing diabetes in some people, but conclusive research isn't available yet.

Age

As we've seen, type 1 diabetes is essentially a disease that strikes the young. The older you get, the higher the risk for developing type 2 diabetes – hence the previously used names 'maturity-onset' and 'adult-onset' diabetes. Most people with the condition are, in fact, diagnosed over the age of 40, while the peak age for diagnosis is around 60. In the industrialised world, between 10 and 20 per cent of people over 65 have type 2.

Unfortunately, the epidemic of obesity, unhealthy eating and sedentary lifestyles now gripping the West means that type 2 diabetes has been seen in children as young as 13.

Obesity

As we have now seen abundantly, if you're obese, you should be aware that this is a major risk factor for type 2 diabetes. Compared to people in the healthy weight range for their height, an obese man is seven times more likely to develop type 2, while an obese woman is an astonishing 27 times more likely to do so.

In fact, the greatest risk factor for developing type 2 diabetes is 'apple-shape' obesity, in which excess fat is stored around the midriff. This pattern of fat storage is seen much more often in men, but is now becoming more common in women, too.

Visceral fat: why 'apple shapes' are risky

The so-called 'visceral' fat packed around your internal organs is more active in terms of cell metabolism than fat stored under your skin. Visceral fat is not just an inert blob of lard; it makes powerful chemicals and hormones, too. In particular, it releases more of a type of fat known as non-esterified fatty acids (NEFAs), which are thought to cause insulin resistance (see page 4), to stimulate the production of glucose in the liver, and to reduce the amount of glucose taken up into muscle cells and used as fuel. These factors lead to reduced (or sometimes increased) insulin secretion and higher glucose levels – and as a result, significantly up the risk of developing type 2 diabetes.

For more information about the link between obesity, diabetes and metabolic syndrome, see Chapter 4.

Activity levels

Your day-to-day level of activity is a real factor in diabetes. If you use your car all the time instead of walking, play no sports, shun the gym and have, bit by bit, adopted the 'couch potato' lifestyle that's become so prevalent, you significantly increase your risk of developing type 2 diabetes. The reason is that exercise increases the sensitivity of muscle cells to insulin. Slim people who exercise regularly are almost five times less likely to develop diabetes than overweight people who lead sedentary lives.

More information on why regular exercise can prevent diabetes may be found in Appendix 1.

Diagnosis

The route to diagnosis can be long, and involve a lot of detours. You may be overweight, and/or experiencing unusual thirst, a constant urge to urinate, and some of the other symptoms listed on pages 6–8, and go to the doctor suspecting it might be diabetes.

Or, feeling odd or 'under the weather', you may have visited your doctor, who – putting two and two together – may decide to test you. Or you may be tested as part of a routine check-up. In any case, here's a rundown of the kind of tests you may have to undergo. They are all simple, and relatively quick.

Urine tests

Your doctor may first use urine testing, the results of which may alert them to the need for further testing. A sample of your urine is checked for sugar with a simple glucose-sensitive dip-stick. Glucose only usually reaches the urine – via seepage from filtered blood through the kidneys – when levels in the blood reach the so-called 'renal threshold'. The average renal threshold occurs at a blood glucose level of 10mmol/l, but the range is wide, at 7 to 13mmol/l. A urine test for glucose is therefore not conclusive, and measuring blood glucose levels is a much more accurate way of diagnosing diabetes.

Blood glucose tests

The results of a blood glucose test depend on whether or not you have eaten. A so-called 'non-fasting' or 'random' blood glucose test can be carried out, but this may show higher blood glucose levels if you have recently eaten a carbohydrate-rich meal. So it's best to have a 'fasting' blood glucose test first thing in the morning, before you have eaten. This will give the most accurate measurement of how well your body handles sugar.

Further testing

Depending on the results of your blood glucose test, your doctor may or may not decide to test further. Early criteria based on an international consensus on diabetes, introduced by the World Health Organization in 1980, suggested that in people with classic diabetes symptoms and signs and a substantially raised blood glucose level – that is, above 15mmol/l – a diagnosis of diabetes could be made without further testing. If the blood glucose level is intermediate (8 to 15mmol/l), however, the criteria suggest referring the person for an oral glucose tolerance test (OGTT).

In 1997, the American Diabetes Association suggested modifying the WHO's criteria by lowering the fasting blood glucose level at which diabetes is diagnosed to 7mmol/l. The ADA guidelines suggest that diabetes can be diagnosed if:

- a person has classic symptoms, plus a random blood glucose level greater than, or equal to, 11.1mmol/l, OR
- a fasting blood glucose showing a level greater than, or equal to, 7mmol/l, OR
- an oral glucose tolerance test shows a blood glucose level greater than, or equal to, 11.1mmol/l two hours after drinking a 75g glucose solution.

Your fasting blood glucose level will usually be confirmed the day after testing, to doublecheck the result.

The ADA criteria also define a fasting glucose level as 'impaired' if it is between 6.1 and 7.0mmol/l. It is estimated that every year, up to 5 per cent of people with impaired glucose tolerance go on to develop true diabetes. But some who are retested are shown to have reverted to normal glucose tolerance – especially if they have heeded the warning and made appropriate changes to their diet and lifestyle.

If you've been diagnosed

A diagnosis of diabetes can be a big shock, and you may be feeling anything from confusion to high anxiety. But be assured: you have more control over diabetes than you might think. Those shifts in diet and lifestyle really do make a difference.

If you or your child has type 1 diabetes, a top-notch diet, certain carefully chosen supplements and insulin can help you manage the condition highly efficiently. And if it is type 2, it can be possible – given how well you stick to the changes I recommend – to stop taking pills or even injecting insulin, although you must only ever do this with the full permission and support of your GP or specialist. I outline everything you'll need to do starting with Chapter 4. But first, let's look at the increasingly widespread condition known as metabolic syndrome, which can be a precursor to full-blown type 2 diabetes.

Metabolic syndrome
....

Metabolic syndrome is on the rise and very much in the news. In the US, 24 per cent of the population are estimated to have it, while in the UK and Denmark the figures are 20 per cent and 16 per cent, respectively. But what, exactly, is this condition?

Also known as syndrome X or Reaven's syndrome – after Gerald Reaven, the doctor who first recognised it in the late 1980s – metabolic syndrome is actually a cluster of risk factors, the main ones being obesity, high blood pressure, high levels of triglycerides (a type of blood fat), low levels of 'good' cholesterol and high blood sugar. We'll look at these, and others, in more detail below.

Metabolic syndrome is sometimes called 'prediabetes', as it makes sufferers much more likely to develop type 2 diabetes. And like type 2 diabetes itself, the syndrome is linked with inherited genes, and diet and lifestyle factors such as eating excessive amounts of refined carbohydrates and failing to exercise enough.

Interlocking symptoms

The basis: insulin resistance The underlying cause of metabolic syndrome is insulin resistance. This can be an inherited condition – you may have inherited genes that affect the production of insulin and/or the cell receptors that detect its presence. Or, as we've seen, it can result when you eat too many sugary or refined carbohydrates over a long period of time. Those floods of glucose into the blood trigger repeated floods of insulin.

Eventually, your body's cells fail to respond properly to the hormone – in other words, they become insulin resistant. This causes your pancreas to make yet more insulin to help push all that excess glucose into your muscle and fat cells. This can lead to overweight and obesity, particularly around the midriff (see box below). And in a particularly nasty twist, obesity – a classic sign of metabolic syndrome – can in its turn lead to further deterioration in insulin sensitivity.

Insulin and obesity

When insulin allows glucose to enter your muscle cells, it is used as a fuel or is converted into glycogen – a starchy storage form – for future use. In fat cells, however, insulin promotes the conversion of glucose into triglycerides, a type of blood fat, for storage. It also stops the release of free fatty acids and glycerol (both components of triglycerides) from your fat stores by inhibiting an enzyme, hormone-sensitive lipase, which is needed to mobilise fat before it can be released and burned for energy. Your fat cells respond to lower levels of insulin than your muscle cells, so insulin largely works to move glucose out of the bloodstream into fat stores – and, as it stops the release of fat from your fat cells, insulin actively promotes overweight and obesity (see page 53).

People with metabolic syndrome are basically overdosing on glucose and insulin, and develop a number of symptoms as a result, including difficulty losing weight, tiredness all the time and sugar cravings – the so-called vicious circle of metabolic syndrome.

The rest of the risk factors In addition to insulin resistance, high insulin levels, overweight and obesity (especially of the apple-shape variety), the other clinical findings metabolic syndrome is associated with include:
- high blood pressure
- impaired glucose tolerance (levels of blood glucose that are high, but not as high as in diabetes)
- high levels of 'bad' cholesterol – the very low density lipoprotein variety (VLDL-cholesterol)
- low levels of 'good' cholesterol – HDL cholesterol
- high levels of triglycerides in the bloodstream, especially after meals
- increased blood clotting factors, making blood more sticky.

All these separate conditions are important independent risk factors for heart disease and stroke, and recent evidence suggests that they are 'more than the sum of their parts' – they interact to produce more damage to artery walls than might be expected from their additive effects alone.

There is now evidence, for instance, that raised levels of insulin, as happens in insulin resistance, encourage hardening and furring up of your arteries (a condition known as atherosclerosis) by stimulating the growth, proliferation and movement of smooth muscle cells in artery linings, as well as increasing the uptake of LDL cholesterol into artery walls. Excess insulin can also increase blood pressure, which in turn damages artery linings, and may increase blood stickiness and abnormal clotting processes.

Metabolic syndrome has therefore been described as a 'cardiovascular time-bomb'.

But as it is a precursor to type 2 diabetes, the syndrome can also be seen as a useful guidepost to help identify people at risk of developing both that, and cardiovascular disease, giving them the time to adjust and make the right dietary and lifestyle changes.

Diagnosing metabolic syndrome

As it is typically a cluster of symptoms and signs, metabolic syndrome is only diagnosed when three or more of these risk factors are present. There is no consensus as yet on diagnosis, but in 1999 the European Group for the Study of Insulin Resistance suggested the following definition (measurements described as 'fasting' are made before food first thing in the morning):

- fasting blood insulin levels in the highest 25 per cent for any one population

PLUS any two of the following:
- central (apple-shape) obesity with a high waist measurement greater than or equal to 94cm in men and 80cm in women
- glucose levels greater than or equal to 6.1mmol/l (but less than 7.0mmol/l which would indicate diabetes)
- abnormal blood fat levels (high fasting triglyceride levels of greater than 2.0mmol/l, or HDL cholesterol of less than 1.0mmol/l)
- high blood pressure greater than 140/90mmHg.

This looks a daunting list. But as you'll see in later chapters, my recommendations for healthy eating, an active lifestyle and effective supplements constitute the best natural way of balancing your blood glucose levels and bringing your weight under control – moves that will bring with them a cascade of beneficial effects, including the lowering of your triglyceride levels and blood pressure. And this lifestyle is also the best way of preventing a slide into type 2 diabetes.

From the cardiovascular point of view, there is excellent evidence that if you improve single risk factors such as high blood pressure, raised glucose levels or abnormal cholesterol levels, you can reduce your risk of a heart attack or stroke. A number of researchers, in fact, are interested in whether making aggressive diet and lifestyle changes at an early stage in the development of metabolic syndrome, and even using anti-obesity drugs, might prevent the development of these major risk factors altogether. To date, weight loss is the only intervention that has been shown to improve all of the cardiovascular risk factors seen in people with metabolic syndrome.

See Chapter 4 for a detailed discussion of how to lower your risk of developing metabolic syndrome and type 2 diabetes.

2

Long-term complications

Diabetes need never stop you from having a full and wonderful life. The key here is managing the disease well, and the first step in that process is accepting that you have a serious condition. Then, you need to commit yourself to following the treatment your doctor prescribes – as well as the simple rules for healthy living I outline in this book. If you underestimate the condition or fail to modify any poor health habits you may have picked up over the years (drinking too much alcohol, smoking, lack of exercise), you can put yourself at risk of developing a number of long-term complications.

The information in this chapter is not meant to frighten. It simply lays out the facts, so you know what you'll be avoiding by taking optimal care of yourself.

It is vitally important, above all, to keep your blood glucose levels consistent, between 4 and 7mmol/l (see page 47). If your glucose levels are persistently higher than this, you will dramatically increase your risk of developing complications.

The people most at risk of complications will usually have had diabetes for over a decade, be obese, or will fail to achieve tight, long-term blood glucose control. The stakes are high: if you're not assiduous in managing this condition, your life expectancy falls by around 25 per cent.

But there is tremendous good news. As you'll see when we discuss potential complications, there are a range of approaches available to treat them. I expand on the natural treatments mentioned later in the book.

Why high glucose levels are harmful

In diabetes, as you've learned, your blood glucose levels are persistently raised. When this happens, glucose interacts with proteins in your circulation to form sugar-protein complexes. This process, glycosylation, is very damaging to cells. Your metabolism will also become abnormal and generate large amounts of 'free radicals' – atoms or molecules formed from the process of combustion, including the 'burning' of fuel in your own body (see page 123).

Both these sugar-protein complexes and free radicals are harmful, and can damage blood vessels throughout your body. Damage to large blood vessels increases the risk of hardening and furring up of the arteries – atherosclerosis – which in turn increases the risk of high blood pressure, coronary heart diseases such as angina or heart attack, stroke, impotence, ulceration of the legs, gangrene and amputation as well as several different types of dementia, including Alzheimer's. This damage develops more quickly if your blood pressure spirals out of control, if you smoke or if you have abnormal blood levels of cholesterol, triglycerides or the amino acid homocysteine (see page 152). If you have type 2 diabetes, high glucose levels and insulin resistance can also lead to abnormal blood fat levels (especially triglycerides) that increase your risk of complications.

While raised blood glucose levels damage small blood vessels throughout your body, three sites are particularly vulnerable: your retinas, which are the light-sensitive tissue at the back of your eyes that sends images through the optic nerve to the brain; your kidneys, especially the filtering units known as glomeruli; and the sheaths surrounding your nerve fibres, which are made of a fatty substance known as myelin.

The importance of glucose control

A study in 1993, involving 1440 people and known as the Diabetes Control and Complications Trial, showed without doubt that people with type 1 diabetes who follow an intensive treatment regime had much better glucose control and less risk of developing complications than people following a traditional management regime.

The intensive regime involved three or more daily insulin injections or continuous subcutaneous insulin infusion, plus frequent blood glucose self-monitoring to adjust insulin dose, monthly clinic visits, weekly telephone calls and a diet and exercise programme. The traditional regime entailed once or twice daily insulin injection, three-monthly clinic visits, and no adjustment of insulin dose according to blood glucose monitoring.

Over a nine-year period, the intensive treatment regime lowered the risk of eye damage (retinopathy, see page 24) by up to 75 per cent, and also reduced the development of nerve problems.

Similarly, the UK Prospective Diabetes Study of 1998, which involved 3867 people newly diagnosed with type 2 diabetes, showed that those given an intensive treatment regime (a sulphonylurea drug, which increases insulin secretion, or insulin itself, started immediately) did better than those treated conventionally (diet initially, with a sulphonylurea or insulin only added in if control was poor). The intensive regime reduced the risk of complications such as retinopathy by 25 per cent. Those who also kept their blood pressure under control did better than those whose control was less good. A number of nutritional approaches can complement these intensive medical approaches to treatment, and help to improve complications if they do develop.

The main complications

We have seen how too much glucose circulating in your bloodstream can, if uncontrolled, damage many parts of the body. The complications of diabetes range from mild to lethal, and include:
- eye disease
- kidney disease
- nerve problems
- high blood pressure
- coronary heart disease
- stroke
- dementia
- peripheral vascular disease
- foot problems
- erectile dysfunction, including impotence
- diabetic ketoacidosis
- hyperglycaemic coma.

In the sections that follow, we'll be looking at each complication separately – its symptoms, dangers, and treatments both natural and traditional. Note that all the supplements and herbal remedies I list under each condition are discussed fully starting with Chapter 7, which also gives you guidance on usual doses. Do follow the instructions of your nutritional therapist, however, as doses can vary depending on your individual needs.

There are also a handful of conditions that are linked specifically to metabolic syndrome and type 2 diabetes; these are discussed at the end of this chapter.

Eye disease

Symptoms and risks Regular eye examinations are essential when you have diabetes, as the condition can affect your vision in a number of ways. High blood glucose levels affect the water balance of your lens – the transparent structure at the front of the eye that focuses light. This can cause blurred vision, and also accelerates the formation of cataracts, which develop 10 to 15 years earlier than average in people with diabetes. Damage to the blood vessels in your retina can harm your vision or even cause blindness if it affects the macula (the part of the retina responsible for fine vision) or if it is associated with the growth of new blood vessels, which also increases the risk of glaucoma – raised fluid pressure in the eye. The nerves that control your eye movements can also be damaged by high blood glucose levels.

The retina of your eye is the one area in your body where small blood vessels can be viewed directly. When a specialist examines the back of your eye, using an instrument known as an ophthalmoscope, they look for a number of changes in these small vessels. If they reveal any damage, it is safe to say that small blood vessels throughout your body, including the kidneys and brain, will also have sustained similar damage.

These changes include thickening; small 'blow-outs' known as microaneurysms; leaks of protein-rich fluid through the vessels into surrounding tissues; white areas called 'cotton-wool spots', caused by the raising of underlying nerve fibre layer because of a lack of oxygen; and micro-haemorrhages that produce shapes resembling flames, dots or blots. The blood vessels may resemble a string of beads, form loops, or show abnormal branchings, or may overgrow to produce new branchings in an attempt to improve oxygen delivery to the retina. These new blood vessels lie over the retinal blood vessels, and can rupture when the fluid of the eye – the vitreous gel – contracts. In advanced cases, the retina can tear or detach and glaucoma can develop, while damage to the optic nerve and the macula can all lead to loss of vision.

This condition, known as diabetic retinopathy, is one of the leading causes of blindness in the Western world. If you have diabetes, you need to be aware that eye complications are extremely common after you have had the condition for more than 20 years.

Natural treatments Here, prevention is vital, and good control of both glucose levels and blood pressure can help stave off eye and other complications. Laser therapy can treat some complications in the eyes, such as the overgrowth of new blood vessels, macular damage and potential detachment of the retina.

You can also take a number of supplements to help protect your eyes. These include:
• vitamin C
• vitamin E
• carotenoids such as lutein
• Pycnogenol® (a powerful antioxidant derived from maritime pine bark)
• B group vitamins
• bilberry
• Ginkgo.

Drugs and other treatments Interestingly, even if you have diabetes and normal blood pressure, treatment with an anti-hypertensive drug (an ACE-inhibitor such as lisinopril) can still markedly reduce your risk of developing retinopathy.

Kidney disease

Symptoms and risks Kidney disease due to diabetes is known as diabetic nephropathy. This is a serious condition, as kidneys do a range of vital jobs in the body – filtering blood, producing certain hormones, getting rid of waste and excess water, and even helping to regulate the manufacture of red blood cells.

Diabetes can affect your kidneys in several ways. Hardening and furring up of small arteries supplying blood to the kidneys' filtration units can reduce blood supply to your kidneys, damaging their ability to function properly. High blood glucose levels meanwhile can encourage urinary tract infections, which can lead to scarring in the kidneys.

Over time, raised glucose levels can damage your kidney's filtration units, the glomeruli, thickening their lining. This process can start within two years of developing diabetes, and can eventually reduce the amount of liquid your kidneys are capable of filtering.

The first sign that you have kidney damage is usually the presence of proteins in your urine, as the thickened glomeruli become leaky and allow albumin, a blood protein, to pass through. At the same time, they may fail to filter out waste products. After 20 years of having type 1 diabetes, about one in three people will have protein in the blood, a condition known as proteinuria. Your doctor can test you for this using a simple urine dipstick.

Once protein is persistently present in the urine, your kidney function will usually slowly decrease. Urine production falls, and in two out of three people kidney failure may result.

Natural treatments You can help to reduce the risk of developing diabetic nephropathy by keeping your blood pressure and blood glucose well balanced. Controlling the factors associated with circulatory damage is also important, so you will need to control your levels of bad cholesterol and the amino acid homocysteine, lose weight if you are overweight or obese, and up your activity levels. These measures can both reduce your risk of developing kidney disease, or slow its progression if you have it already. Your doctor may recommend you modify your diet and eat less protein.

A number of nutritional supplements can help protect your kidneys, including:
• alpha-lipoic acid (ALA), a powerful antioxidant
• B group vitamins.

Drugs and other treatments For those with type 2 diabetes, switching over to insulin treatment rather than oral drugs is usually suggested. When kidney function deteriorates significantly, you will need dialysis. Eventually, you may have to consider a kidney transplant.

Nerve problems

Symptoms and risks Diabetes can damage the fatty myelin sheath surrounding your nerve fibres, which in turn slows down your nerve signals. This is known as diabetic neuropathy, and often starts with burning or stinging sensations in areas supplied by affected nerves. As a result, you may find it harder to sense vibration, pain or extremes of temperature – especially in your feet. Risk arises when a cut or blister goes unnoticed; a small injury may become ulcerated and infection may set in, exacerbated by poor circulation and raised glucose levels. A related symptom is restless legs – in which there is an unpleasant creeping sensation in the lower limbs, accompanied by twitching, pins and needles, burning sensations or pain plus an irresistible urge to move the legs.

Neuropathy can also cause weakness or wasting of your muscles, and deformities such as 'hammer' toes (where a toe assumes a claw-like position, a condition that can lead to ulceration), and can contribute to impotence in men.

Natural treatments Research involving people with both type 1 and type 2 diabetes has shown that good long-term control of blood glucose levels can reduce the risk of developing diabetic neuropathy. But if you have it, you will want relief, as it can be a maddeningly painful condition.

Treatment with simple painkillers such as aspirin, paracetamol or codeine phosphate is usually unhelpful, but some people find relief with a cream containing extract of chilli pepper (capsaicin), which reduces the signals sent from pain nerve fibres in the treated area. You can obtain this on prescription from your doctor. Bed cradles to lift bed clothes off the feet may also help.

Leg cramping, an occasional side effect of neuropathy, can sometimes be helped via magnetic therapy, which improves blood flow to affected areas, and boosts oxygenation. An alternative treatment worth considering for restless legs is co-enzyme Q10 (see page 136).

A number of nutritional supplements can help to improve diabetic neuropathy. These include:
• ALA
• B group vitamins, including biotin
• evening primrose oil.

Drugs and other treatments Antidepressants, which affect levels of certain chemicals in the brain, often help to reduce pain perception, especially burning sensations. Shooting pains, often described as like electric shocks, may be reduced by anticonvulsant drugs such as carbamazepine or phenytoin.

Restless legs may be helped by the benzodiazepine drug, clonazepam. Cramping in the leg muscles may be helped by quinine sulphate tablets.

High blood pressure

Symptoms and risks If you have diabetes, you are twice as likely to develop high blood pressure as someone without diabetes. Between 10 and 30 per cent of people with type 1 diabetes, and 30 to 60 per cent of people with type 2, have high blood pressure.

Diabetic nephropathy (see page 25) is thought to contribute to the problem because when excess fluid and salts from the body are not filtered out, they build up in the circulation, and this will raise blood pressure. Kidney disease may also boost secretion of the hormone renin, which is problematic, as it is involved in regulating blood pressure.

In type 1 diabetes, blood pressure usually starts to rise when protein is detectable in the urine (see page 26), while in type 2 high blood pressure is more closely linked to insulin resistance, obesity and the development of abnormal blood fat levels.

In combination, diabetes and high blood pressure have a very damaging effect on your circulation, and are a strong risk factor for coronary heart disease. Having both also increases the risk of small blood vessel complications. In the UK Prospective Diabetes Study of 1998, 1148 people with type 2 diabetes and hypertension were either put on strictly controlled regimes for lowering blood pressure (so their average blood pressure over nine years was 144/82mmHg) or less strictly controlled ones (so their average blood pressure over nine years was 154/87mmHg). Those with the stricter regime were 44 per cent less likely to have a stroke and 37 per cent less likely to develop diabetic eye disease and kidney problems.

Natural treatments If you are diagnosed with high blood pressure, it is vital to make the necessary diet and lifestyle changes. If you smoke, you need to stop; if you're overweight, you will need to lose the excess; and if you are too liberal with salt and alcohol, you will have to cut your consumption of both. Both increasing your activity levels, and learning relaxation techniques, are also crucial when tackling hypertension. It's so important to control blood pressure when you have diabetes that some recommend keeping your blood pressure consistently lower than 130/80mmHg if your kidney function is normal, or less than 125/75mmHg when there is more than 1g protein per 24 hours in the urine. To achieve these targets, it's usually necessary to take more than one antihypertensive drug.

For more information on high blood pressure, see page 58.

A number of nutritional supplements can help to reduce high blood pressure. These include:
- co-enzyme Q10
- potassium
- antioxidants
- magnesium
- garlic
- omega-3 fish oils.

Coronary heart disease

Symptoms and risks If you have diabetes, you are 2 to 6 times more likely to develop coronary heart disease than someone without diabetes. Coronary heart disease happens when your coronary arteries harden and fur up, starving the heart of oxygen-rich blood. This triggers pain known as angina, which is usually:
- felt behind the chest bone
- tight and crushing – like a bear hug
- described as spreading through the chest and may radiate up into the neck, jaw or down the left arm
- brought on by exertion
- relieved by rest.

If the heart muscle is continually starved of oxygen, some of its cells will die, triggering a heart attack. A heart attack feels something like angina, but lasts longer, is more intense, can come on at any time and is unrelieved by rest. It is usually accompanied by sweating, paleness and breathlessness.

Sudden chest pain should always be taken seriously and medical assistance sought without delay. It is important to know, however, that the perception of pain in the heart may not be as acute in people with diabetes, perhaps because of damage to the nerves supplying the heart. So if someone with diabetes develops malaise, sweats, experiences shortness of breath and feels faint, a heart attack should always be suspected, even if they do not have chest pain. Be aware that these symptoms are similar to those of a hypoglycaemic attack, so if it is a heart attack, the diagnosis may be delayed as a result.

Coronary heart disease is particularly common in people with type 2 diabetes. The risk of developing heart problems is higher if, in addition to diabetes, you have high blood pressure, abnormally raised cholesterol levels and a raised homocysteine level (see page 152), and smoke, are overweight and take little exercise.

People with diabetes are also more likely to develop a heart muscle problem known as cardiomyopathy, in which the chambers of the heart do not contract to pump blood as efficiently as normal. Eventually this condition can lead to heart failure.

Natural treatments Strict control of blood glucose levels is vitally important for someone who has diabetes and coronary heart disease.

A number of nutritional supplements can also help atherosclerosis and coronary heart disease. These include:
- vitamin C
- vitamin E
- co-enzyme Q10
- tea (green, black, white or oolong)
- selenium
- B group vitamins
- chromium
- copper
- magnesium
- garlic
- omega-3 fish oils
- evening primrose oil.

Drugs and other treatments Among the drugs used to treat coronary heart disease are aspirin (which reduces blood clotting), beta-blockers (which slow heart rate to reduce heart work load), ACE inhibitors (which have several actions that reduce the workload of the heart) and statins (which lower cholesterol levels). If you have type 2 diabetes and coronary heart disease, be aware that if you're not already using insulin you may be switched to it.

Stroke

Symptoms and risks A stroke happens when there is a sudden interruption of blood supply to part of the brain, leading to a loss of control of one or more body parts or functions. People with diabetes are two to four times more likely to have a stroke than people without diabetes.

There are three main types of stroke: a thrombosis, in which a clot forms in a brain artery (45 per cent of cases); an embolism, in which a clot forms elsewhere in the circulation and travels in the bloodstream to lodge in the brain (35 per cent), or a haemorrhage, in which a ruptured blood vessel causes bleeding within or over the surface of the brain (20 per cent).

A so-called 'mini-stroke' can also occur, where symptoms fully resolve within 24 hours. Known as a transient ischaemic attack (TIA), this kind of stroke is thought to happen when small clumps of blood platelets lodge within the brain to temporarily block the circulation to some brain cells. The platelet clots break up and clear before brain cells die from lack of oxygen, however. A TIA is an important warning sign that a stroke may occur in the future. If TIAs are treated (say, by taking a drug that lowers platelet stickiness), a full-blown stroke can often be prevented

Natural treatments A stroke can kill or disable, so prevention is very important. Some research suggests that people with a good intake of vitamin C are half as likely to suffer a stroke as those with an intake of less than 28mg of the vitamin a day. It may seem astonishing, but drinking a glass of orange or grapefruit juice every day may significantly reduce your risk of stroke by as much as 25 per cent!

The Stroke Association encourages people to eat five to six portions of fruit and vegetables a day, as this can reduce the risk of stroke by up to 30 per cent. Even if you don't manage that much, increasing your usual intake by just one serving per day has been shown to lower the risk of a stroke by around 6 per cent (in people without diabetes). Tight glucose control remains vitally important, too, which may influence your choice of fruit and vegetables (see page 84).

A number of nutritional supplements can help to reduce the risk of stroke, and are also beneficial if you have previously experienced a stroke. These include:
- vitamin C
- B group vitamins.

Drugs and other treatments Someone who has had a stroke may require varying amounts of support. Some people may be managed at home, while others need intensive care. In some cases, specific treatment is needed, such as aspirin to reduce the formation of tiny platelet clots, or a clot-busting (thrombolytic) drug to dissolve a larger clot. Physiotherapy, speech therapy and occupational therapy will help to restore lost movement, speech disturbance and help with rehabilitation.

Dementia

Symptoms and risks Dementia currently affects over 700,000 people in the UK. The most common form is Alzheimer's disease (AD) which affects an estimated 385,000 people. Because we are an ageing population, it is estimated that by the year 2010, there will be about 462,000 people with Alzheimer's dementia in the UK, rising to over 825,000 people by 2050.

The exact cause of dementia remains unknown. It probably results from a combination of different factors such as increasing age, diet, environmental factors and the genes you have inherited which result in progressive destruction of brain cells.

The first symptoms of dementia are usually mild forgetfulness when trying to remember recent events or the names of friends, family or familiar things. Longer term memory for childhood events may be unaffected, however. It may also become difficult solving simple sums or finding the right words to describe what you mean. Although these symptoms are often normal in older people, and in those who are over-worked or stressed, in someone with dementia the symptoms become noticeably worse with time, and disorientation and confusion start to cause concern. Problems with self care, confusion, speaking, reading, thinking and carrying out the normal activities of daily living eventually develop and this can understandably lead to anxiety, mood swings and sometimes aggressiveness. Eventually, someone with dementia will need total care and attention.

Natural treatments Some research suggests that increasing your intake of folic acid may help to protect against Alzheimer's disease. Folic acid is needed to make some brain chemicals, but its protective role probably comes from its ability to lower blood levels of the amino acid, homocysteine (see page 152) which is linked with several forms of dementia. People with raised levels of homocysteine appear to be twice as likely to develop Alzheimer's as those with low levels.

Some researchers have found that taking vitamin E may help to slow the progress of some symptoms of AD for a limited time.

Herbal extracts from Ginkgo biloba leaves improve blood flow to the brain and may help to improve memory in some people with Alzheimer's disease.

Drugs and other treatments Unfortunately, there is no treatment that can cure or prevent the progression of dementia, although drugs known as cholinesterase inhibitors (e.g. donepezil, rivastigmine galantamine) are available for those with mild or moderate Alzheimer's disease (AD). These drugs help to prevent the breakdown of a brain chemical called acetylcholine which is involved in memory and thought, and some people with dementia who take a cholinesterase inhibitor drug notice an improvement in their ability to think, and it may help stop symptoms worsening for a limited time.

Recently, it was thought that inflammation in the brain may contribute to AD and scientists are investigating whether non-steroidal anti-inflammatory drugs (NSAIDs related to aspirin) might help to slow the progression of AD, although they do not appear to help people who already have advanced symptoms.

Peripheral vascular disease

Symptoms and risks If your arteries become progressively more hardened and furred up, this can reduce blood flow to your extremities, resulting in peripheral vascular disease. This condition is four times more common in people with diabetes than in those without the disease.

The legs are most affected in peripheral vascular disease. Because blood flow is reduced, you may experience pain in your calves while exercising (intermittent claudication); while the lack of oxygen and nutrients to tissues can lead to ulceration of the legs. If your blood vessels become completely closed, tissues may die and become infected, allowing gangrene to set in. Peripheral vascular disease can also contribute towards impotence (see page 36).

Natural treatments Controlling your blood glucose, blood pressure and blood cholesterol levels is the best prevention against the arterial hardening and furring up that leads to peripheral vascular disease. Keeping blood levels of homocysteine (see page 152) right down is also important, as this amino acid is also linked to circulatory problems.

A number of nutritional supplements can help peripheral vascular disease. These include:
• vitamin C
• B group vitamins
• bilberry
• garlic
• Ginkgo.

Foot problems

Symptoms and risks The most common reason for people with diabetes being admitted to hospital is some kind of problem with the feet, such as ulcers. Diabetic neuropathy or nerve problems (see page 27), poor blood supply and infection that spreads may all cause foot ulcers.

Nerve problems boost the risk of developing foot ulcers in several ways. An abnormal nerve supply to the foot muscles can lead to high arches, clawed toes or hammer toe, which produce uneven pressure while walking. Reduced sensation in the feet can also mean people tend to walk more heavily. Any of these changes may boost the formation of calluses, rubbing and tissue damage which, because of reduced sensation, may not be noticed. In time, continued pressure can lead to ulceration.

As we've seen, having diabetes means that your skin's healing ability is reduced due to poor blood supply, as your tissues receive less oxygen and nutrients than they need. So detecting foot ulceration at an early stage is extremely important. If not treated early and thoroughly, it can lead to spreading infection of soft tissues (cellulitis), abscess, infection of the underlying bone (osteomyelitis), blood poisoning (septicaemia) or gangrene. These complications may require the amputation of toes, the foot or part of the leg below the knee. It is unfortunate, but people with diabetes are 16 times more likely to need a leg amputation than someone without diabetes.

Natural treatments Because a tiny wound can potentially escalate into an amputation, this is another case where prevention is all-important. If you have diabetes, looking after your feet carefully is a big priority. Check them daily for signs of redness, blisters, cuts or other wounds such as athlete's foot. If this is difficult, ask a friend or relative to check for you so that any signs of infection or inflammation can be reported immediately. Foot ulcers tend to develop at pressure points on the underside of the feet, over the heads of the metatarsal bones (just below where the toes join the foot), on the big toe or at the heel. Ulcers can also occur on the tips or tops of the toes, between the toes or on the sides of the foot due to improperly fitting shoes.

A number of supplements can help diabetic foot ulcers, including:
• magnesium
• aloe vera
• zinc.

Garlic powder tablets and Ginkgo biloba supplements will improve blood flow through tiny blood vessels, which will in turn boost blood circulation in the base of the ulcer and encourage healing. Include oily fish such as wild salmon, sardines, mackerel or herrings in your weekly menus or take fish oil supplements, as this will help to thin the blood and promote healing of leg ulcers.

Drugs and other treatments If you develop a foot ulcer, it is vitally important to control your blood sugar levels, and to prevent complications resulting from the poor circulation of blood to your feet. Good hygiene is essential, as otherwise there is a danger that infection might make amputation necessary. You will be advised to wash your feet daily with mild soap or a saline solution, and to keep the ulcer covered with clean, dry dressings.

Care of the ulcer will usually be overseen by a nurse attached to your GP practice, and you may even have to have complete bed rest. Antibiotics will be needed at the first sign of infection. Interesting new research suggests that using maggots to clear away dead tissue is surprisingly beneficial, helping to clean the wound and allow it to heal faster than with conventional treatment. However, this treatment is not routinely available and its provision will depend on the individual interests of the consultants in your area. The use of medical honeys to help wounds heal is also increasing in popularity.

Erectile dysfunction and impotence

Symptoms and risks Diabetes is a major cause of erectile difficulties in men. Up to a quarter of all males with diabetes aged 30 to 34 are affected, increasing to 75 per cent of those aged 60 to 64 years. Some reports suggest that impotence eventually affects around one in two men with diabetes. But as you will see below, there are now a number of effective treatments for the condition, and the all-important task of controlling glucose levels over the long term should make any problems with getting or maintaining an erection less likely to develop in the first place.

Poorly controlled diabetes is linked with impotence because persistently raised blood glucose levels affect both circulation to the penis (by hastening furring up of the arteries) and its nerve supply (reducing sensation and affecting nerve signals needed to control the onset of erections). The side effects of drugs used to treat co-existing conditions such as high blood pressure and heart problems may also contribute to the problem.

Not surprisingly, impotence has a serious effect on a couple's relationship. Over 20 per cent of men with erectile dysfunction blame it for the break-up of their relationships, yet many men avoid seeking help due to embarrassment or a fear that tests will be invasive or uncomfortable.

In most cases, however, only simple questions and a brief physical examination are involved, and often the only investigations needed are measuring blood pressure and simple urinary and blood tests. A number of options for treatment are now available for the condition, including supplements and some very promising new drugs and other treatments.

Natural treatments A number of nutritional supplements can help to improve erectile dysfunction, including:
• vitamin C
• co-enzyme Q10
• Ginkgo
• ginseng.

Drugs and other treatments The treatment of impotence has been revolutionised with the advent of new therapies such as locally acting medications (including urethral pellets of alprostadil) and oral tablets such as sildenafil (Viagra), tadalafil (Cialis), vardenafil (Levitra) and apomorphine (Uprima).

Where drugs are ineffectual or inadvisable because of health problems, mechanical aids (vacuum devices and penile implants) are available. Vascular surgery to bypass blockages in arterial blood flow to the penis, or correct leaking veins that allow too much blood to drain away from the penis during erection, is also possible. As a result, more than 9 out of 10 men with erectile difficulties are able to regain potency with one of the many treatments now available.

Diabetic ketoacidosis

Symptoms and risks If people with type 1 diabetes fail to boost their levels of insulin for any reason, severe and uncontrolled diabetes with dangerously high blood glucose levels can result. Because muscle and fat cells cannot absorb glucose with little or no insulin available, their metabolism becomes abnormal and they have to burn free fatty acids and protein as fuel instead. As a result, acids and ketones – breakdown products of fat – build up in their circulation along with the excess glucose, and they become severely dehydrated, producing a state known as diabetic ketoacidosis. This condition carries a mortality rate of 5 to 10 per cent and is a medical emergency needing immediate treatment in intensive care. It is most common in younger people, but is most dangerous for older people, who are less likely to survive.

Ketoacidosis usually develops in people whose diabetes has not been diagnosed, or in people with established diabetes who are not being treated properly or who develop an infection, which stimulates the release of stress hormones and increases the need for insulin. In many cases, however, no obvious cause is identified. The symptoms and signs of ketoacidosis include:
- excessive thirst and urine production
- dehydration
- 'acetone' smell on the breath
- weakness
- blurred vision
- rapid pulse
- rapid breathing
- abdominal pain (especially in children)
- leg cramping
- weight loss
- nausea and vomiting
- confusion and drowsiness
- low blood pressure
- low temperature.

Treatment If not treated, diabetic ketoacidosis can lead to coma. The treatment involves giving fluids and salts by infusion, plus slow-acting insulin, until blood glucose levels come down. Antibiotics may be needed if infection is suspected.

Hyperglycaemic coma

Symptoms and risks In people with type 2 diabetes, blood glucose levels may rise very high; but they are still producing some insulin, so they do not develop ketoacidosis. Very high blood glucose levels lead to symptoms such as:
- excessive thirst and urine production
- dehydration
- weakness
- blurred vision.

If a person with type 2 diabetes in this state develops an infection, takes prescribed diuretic drugs to reduce fluid retention, or drinks lots of glucose-rich fluids in an attempt to quench their unusually severe thirst, they can slip into a hyperglycaemic coma, which is associated with very high levels of glucose (as opposed to the hypoglycaemic coma, which can result from very low levels of glucose).

Treatment The treatment for hyperglycaemic coma is similar to that for ketoacidosis, and involves rehydration with a fluid and salt infusion plus low-dose insulin until blood glucose levels come down. Antibiotics may be needed if infection is suspected. Afterwards, regular insulin injections are given for a few months, but many people can then switch to following a diet and exercise regime with or without an oral hypoglycaemic drug.

Conditions linked to type 2 diabetes and metabolic syndrome

While the complications listed above are risks with type 1 or severe type 2 diabetes, several diseases are strongly linked to metabolic syndrome and type 2 diabetes. These are listed below.

Fatty liver disease

A build-up of fat in liver cells can cause a condition known as non-alcoholic fatty liver disease (NAFLD). This affects as many as 20 per cent of the population and is so strongly linked with insulin resistance that it has been suggested as a liver manifestation of metabolic syndrome.

A form of liver inflammation known as non-alcoholic steatohepatitis (NASH) is a type of NAFLD, and is also linked with raised insulin levels and insulin resistance. It is not yet known whether NASH is a cause or the result of insulin resistance, but it is likely that insulin resistance in fat cells leads to an increase in the amount of free fatty acids in the bloodstream which, in turn, are taken up by the liver, where they cause inflammation.

Treatment aims to correct underlying risk factors and may

involve taking drugs that help to protect the liver. This is important, as those with liver inflammation are six times more likely to develop liver cirrhosis.

One of the most successful natural approaches to improving NAFLD is to follow a low-carbohydrate diet (outlined in Chapter 6).

Polycystic ovary syndrome

Type 2 diabetes, impaired glucose tolerance and metabolic syndrome in women are all linked with an increased chance of developing the gynaecological condition polycystic ovary syndrome (PCOS). This may be because raised levels of insulin stimulate the production of more male hormones (androgens) than is normal in the ovaries. Women with PCOS may put on weight, grow excess hair, and develop irregular periods.

Working hard to keep blood sugar in balance and following a low-carbohydrate diet constitute the best natural treatment for PCOS.

Medical treatment with the drug metformin (see page 45), which reduces insulin resistance, is also becoming more popular.

Medical management

While eating right, staying fit and boosting your health with effective vitamins, minerals and herbs are vital for your day-to-day management of diabetes, medical treatments and tests may also enter the picture. Procedures such as insulin injections and glucose testing are an essential part of managing type 1, and in some cases insulin or drugs may be needed with type 2 and metabolic syndrome.

So I will be running through the range of medical treatments you may encounter. Depending on the kind and severity of your diabetes, some may – along with diet, exercise and supplementation – go to form the backbone of your daily regime. This chapter also covers treatment for children with type 1 diabetes.

Treatments for type 1 diabetes

When you are diagnosed with type 1 diabetes, your way of life changes. In essence, you must do consciously something your body has done for you up to now: step in for the pancreas, which is unable to produce enough insulin to keep your blood glucose on an even keel. So you will need to inject insulin and, along with people who have type 2, you must also carefully monitor your levels of blood glucose, up to several times a day. (See page 47 for how to keep an eye on your blood glucose levels.)

Insulin treatment

If you are just starting your insulin programme, you will have had instruction from your doctor or clinic nurse, and you'll know what to expect. Yet this doesn't necessarily mean the process won't seem strange at the start – perhaps even intimidating. You may feel burdened by the notion of a lifetime of insulin injections stretching before you, or scared that you'll botch your self-injections. This section aims to demystify the process, which over the past few decades has changed to become much faster and easier.

Why inject? Insulin can't be taken by mouth: it is broken down by digestive juices before it is absorbed. So you will need to inject it. If you feel nervous or squeamish about this process, don't worry – any notion that you will be wielding a huge syringe or experiencing a lot of pain is way off the mark. These days, injections are given through fine needles that hardly sting as they go in. The syringes and so-called 'pens', which incorporate a cartridge, are small and easy to carry and use.

Types of insulin and how to store it Although animal insulin, for example from pigs or cows, is still available, it's far more likely that you will be injecting 'human' insulin manufactured by inserting the relevant gene into bacterial or yeast cultures (or by modifying pig insulin to make it identical to human insulin).

Insulin comes in either clear, or cloudy, forms. The clear is faster-acting, while the cloudy version has a delayed action. Depending on what your doctor decides, you may need to inject one dose of clear insulin before each meal; or you may inject a cloudy insulin once or twice a day. The programme of insulin injections your doctor will recommend aims to mimic the insulin levels that would normally occur in your body. Over time, you and your doctor will need to adjust the frequency of your injections as you get used to the regime and check the pattern of your blood glucose levels.

Your insulin may come in either a self-sealing bottle or a cartridge, and it will have an expiry date. It won't 'go off' under ordinary conditions, but you must protect it from very low or very high temperatures. Keeping it in the fridge at between 2 and 10°C is optimal.

When and how much to inject You will usually need to inject a dose of insulin one to four times a day. The pattern of injection will be determined by your individual needs, and also to mimic the way insulin is secreted naturally.

In people without diabetes, insulin is usually secreted in a quick pulse immediately after a meal (which stimulates the fat and muscle cells to absorb glucose), followed by a slower, more prolonged rise in insulin levels that fall to a steady level between meals and throughout the night. So you will usually need to combine a short-acting insulin to mimic the peak in production after a meal, plus a delayed-action insulin to maintain insulin levels between meals.

Very rapidly acting insulins start to work around 15 minutes after injection, and can be given up to 15 minutes before or after a meal. Their effects last from 2 to 5 hours.

Short-acting insulins (regular or soluble insulins) are fast-acting, and their effects peak between 2 and 4 hours after injection, but last for up to around 8 hours.

Intermediate and long-acting insulins start acting around 1 to 4 hours after injection, and can last up to 35 hours. A new form, insulin glargine, starts to be released 1.5 hours after injection, and diffuses constantly and evenly into the bloodstream over 24 hours. It only needs to be injected once a day. This provides an even blood glucose level throughout the day, with no pronounced highs or lows, which may reduce the risk of hypoglycaemia.

Where to inject The best sites are generally beneath the skin of your upper outer arms, buttocks, lower abdomen or upper outer thighs. Absorption of insulin is fastest from the abdomen and slowest from the buttocks and thighs. You will need to rotate the site of your injections, as otherwise there can be a breakdown or build-up of fat in the injected area

New-generation insulin devices Recent technological advances in the field of insulin delivery include the development of devices that continuously infuse insulin under the skin. This is known as continuous subcutaneous insulin infusion (CSII) and more closely mimics natural patterns of insulin secretion in the body, but it is not for everyone – your doctor will be able to advise you on this. Insulin pumps that can be implanted under the skin are also under development, as are pancreatic islet cell implants.

Treating children with type 1 diabetes

When a youngster has diabetes, the whole family becomes involved. The thought of sticking needles into a young child is naturally horrifying for parents; but young children are remarkably adaptable, and they will soon accept injections as a normal part of their life.

If your child is very young when diagnosed, it can help get them used to the idea of injection to play games, such as injecting teddy with his own needle, or even injecting yourself (without insulin). Many children, even from the age of six, are able to inject themselves under supervision, and fun, colourful, trendy-looking insulin pens are now available. Skin-prick tests to keep an eye on glucose levels are surprisingly painless with today's automatic pricking devices, which are used on the side of a fingertip, heel or earlobe. Get your child involved by offering them some choices – have them pick the injection site, or choose which finger to get a drop of blood from.

It is vital to discuss your child's school's policy about blood testing (such as in the classroom or clinic) and their access to emergency glucose tablets/sugar. Ensure that your child will be able to have lunch and a mid-morning and mid-afternoon snack at a set time. Extra snacks or glucose may also be needed before and after exercise. Make sure the teachers are aware of the symptoms of a hypo (see page 49), know how to treat it and appreciate that a child with a suspected hypo should never be left alone; and ensure the school knows who to contact in an emergency.

Treatments for type 2 diabetes
....

For 10 to 20 per cent of people with type 2 diabetes, diet and exercise alone are enough to keep their blood glucose levels stable. Some people with the condition, however, will also need tablets that either encourage the production of insulin, help the body use insulin more efficiently, reduce production of new glucose in the liver or slow down the rate at which glucose is absorbed from the intestines so the body can handle it more effectively.

A common pattern for someone with type 2 diabetes is to

progress from handling the condition with diet and exercise alone to taking one, two and sometimes three oral drugs to help lower glucose levels, before eventually needing insulin injections instead. A few may need insulin plus the oral drug metformin. However, this traditional approach to treatment may not be as effective in reducing the future development of complications as a more intensive regime in which medication is started straight away (see page 23).

This pattern of having to take additional drugs is not inevitable, however. Switching to a lower-carbohydrate diet and taking some of the supplements mentioned in this book can help to improve glucose control in someone with type 2 diabetes. In many cases, this can reduce your need for medication, but you should never reduce or stop taking any of your drugs without the full permission and supervision of your own doctor.

Hypoglycaemic drugs

The hypoglycaemic, or glucose-lowering, drugs described in the box below all come in pill form. They have certain contraindications and possible side effects; your doctor will inform you of these before prescribing them.

Common drugs used to treat type 2 diabetes

Sulphonylureas

These drugs (which include glibenclamide – known as glyburide in the US – gliclazide, glimepiride, glipizide and gliquidone) stimulate insulin secretion from your beta cells. Some, such as glimepiride, also increase the activity of insulin. A number of these drugs can cause hypoglycaemia. A side effect of taking sulphonylurea drugs can include weight gain, so they are most helpful for people who are not overweight at diagnosis.

Metformin

Metformin is the only available drug in the class known as biguanides. It works by increasing uptake of glucose into muscle cells, as well as

---

reducing production of new glucose in the liver, and reducing the absorption of glucose from the intestines. This lowers high blood glucose levels without increasing insulin levels or causing hypoglycaemia. One possible side effect is lactic acidosis, a build-up of lactic acid in the blood. As this is also a dangerous side effect of kidney problems, metformin cannot be used by people with type 2 diabetes who also have even mild problems with their kidneys.

One of the main benefits of metformin is that it does not cause weight gain, which is why it is the first-line drug of choice for overweight people with type 2. However, it may lead to raised levels of the potentially harmful amino acid homocysteine (see page 152) by interfering with vitamin absorption.[4] In one study, treatment with metformin was shown to reduce levels of folic acid and vitamin B12, resulting in a modest increase in homocysteine levels (see page 157).[5] This is easily treated by taking folic acid supplements, however (see page 152).[6]

Glitazones

These drugs, which include pioglitazone, rosiglitazone and others, increase the sensitivity of muscle and fat cells to insulin so more glucose is taken up into tissues and used as fuel. They also reduce the breakdown of blood triglycerides to produce free fatty acids, which, in turn, means that muscles burn more glucose, and that less glucose is produced by the liver. These drugs are usually prescribed together with metformin or with a sulphonylurea. People taking these drugs must be monitored to ensure they do not develop heart or liver problems. Glitazones can cause weight gain as a side effect.

Meal-time glucose regulators

Like the sulphonylureas, these drugs – which include nateglinide and repaglinide – also stimulate the release of insulin from the beta cells. They have a rapid but short action and are taken just before each main meal whenever and wherever the person chooses. This means they help to increase insulin secretion when it is needed – when glucose levels are highest just after a meal, but not in between meals, so they are less likely to cause hypoglycaemia (see below) than the sulphonylurea drugs.

Acarbose

A so-called alpha-glucosidase inhibitor, acarbose is taken with a meal and works by slowing the absorption of glucose from the intestines.

This is achieved by blocking the action of a digestive enzyme, alpha-glucosidase, which normally breaks down complex carbohydrates into simpler sugars for absorption. Acarbose can cause side effects such as flatulence, bloating, diarrhoea and pain due to the fermentation of unabsorbed carbohydrates in the large intestine. People using acarbose plus a sulphonylurea are advised to carry dextrose tablets with them at all times (rather than sucrose) in case of hypoglycaemia (see below), as acarbose slows the absorption of sucrose.

Assessing blood glucose levels

Everyone with type 1 diabetes, and people with type 2 diabetes who are taking insulin or a hypoglycaemic drug, must measure their blood glucose levels several times a day. Your doctor will specify how frequently you should test, and when. They will also advise you on testing if you have type 2 that you're controlling well with diet and exercise alone. The test you use should ideally assess the glucose levels in your blood, rather than your urine.

The target blood glucose levels for people with diabetes are usually:
• 4 – 7mmol/l before meals
• 4 – 10mmol/l when checked 90 to 120 minutes after a meal
• 7 – 10mmol/l before having a bedtime snack
• 3.5 – 7mmol/ if checked in the middle of the night (around 3 am).

If you're getting it right, your glucose levels will always show up as between 4 to 7mmol/l. This kind of balance will reduce the risk of complications. If your blood glucose levels regularly show up as too high or too low, your doctor will tell you how to increase or reduce your food intake and/or insulin treatment (short-acting and/or delayed-acting insulin) to keep your glucose levels optimally balanced over the long term.

Your daily tests

Today's home blood glucose tests give highly accurate results – as they have to, because they are key to your health. Your doctor will advise you on where to find the supplies you'll need for daily use – lancets or finger-prickers, colour-change strips and meters.

You need a drop of blood each time you test, and a finger is handiest for this, although some people use their earlobes. Single-use sterile lancets or finger-prickers do the job admirably and with little pain. You then place the drop on a colour-change strip as directed in the accompanying instructions. Once you've dropped it on, you need to place the strip in your meter. (Many of today's meters have integral strip dispensers.) You should get a reading within about 15 seconds. Most metres now in use store the readings, but if yours doesn't, you will need to record them in a notepad.

Glucose measuring equipment is thankfully becoming ever less invasive. Lasers for drawing out the blood have been developed, for instance, making that process even less painful. It's a good idea to keep abreast of developments in glucose measuring equipment, as anything that makes these essential daily readings easier is obviously welcome.

Glycosylated haemoglobin and fructosamine tests

Aside from calling your doctor with any relatively urgent problems that arise, it's a good idea to see them regularly – at least four times a year – for a general checkup and special tests that will give 'snapshots' of your glucose control over the last few weeks or months. Note that these tests do not take the place of your daily blood testing.

The glycosylated haemoglobin test looks for levels of a substance that forms when glucose circulating in the bloodstream interacts with the red blood pigment haemoglobin. The main component is HbA1c, and a blood test to measure levels of this substance gives an excellent idea of your glucose control over the previous two to three months. The goal is to maintain the level of glycosylated HbA1c at below 7 per cent.

Or your doctor may administer another test for fructosamine – a substance formed when glucose reacts with the blood protein albumin. The fructosamine test shows how well your control has been over the last two to three weeks.

When things go wrong: hypoglycaemia

It's important to try to keep your blood glucose level over 4mmol/l. If levels fall too low, you may experience a hypo – short for hypo-glycaemia. Hypos are very common, and if you depend on insulin injections you may have several a year. You'll need to learn the first signs of a hypo coming on so you can treat it promptly.

Officially, hypoglycaemia is defined as having a blood glucose level of less than 2.5mmol/l. When you're in the throes of one, you may:
• become very hungry
• feel light-headed or dizzy
• go pale
• sweat
• get palpitations/pounding heart
• develop double vision
• tremble or shake
• have difficulty speaking
• experience nausea
• develop a headache
• become irritable
• feel weak
• have poor co-ordination
• feel drowsy or confused.

A hypo usually results when there is a mismatch between the timing or dose of insulin or other glucose-lowering medication, and the amount of food you have eaten. Exercise or drinking too much alcohol can also bring on a hypo. They become more common, too, the longer you have diabetes – especially type 1 – because awareness of the early warning signs of the condition seems to lessen over time.

Hypoglycaemia must be treated urgently before it leads to loss of consciousness, by ingesting some sugar – glucose, sucrose or dextrose. So if you are dependent on insulin, you'll need to keep glucose tablets with you at all times. Let all your friends, colleagues and/or teachers know that you'll need sugar in these circumstances, and that they will have to seek medical advice if you start acting oddly, seem 'sleepy' or actually collapse.

If you start feeling your concentration slipping or that you're slowing down or weakening; if you begin craving something sugary like a lolly, yet feel revolted by the idea of food; if your vision blurs; if you start feeling highly emotional 'out of the blue' – in short, if you begin experiencing one or more of the symptoms listed above – you must take this as the first sign of a hypoglycaemic attack. You need to take action right away. (Note that the early warning signs of hypoglycaemia may be less pronounced in people using 'human' insulin than in those using insulins produced from an animal source.)

If you're able to swallow, you should have a carbohydrate-containing drink (*not* the diet version) such as lemonade or cola, and/or take glucose/dextrose tablets. You should follow this by eating a longer-acting source of carbohydrate such as a slice of bread. Instruct friends and loved ones that if you appear unable to swallow, they should smear jam on your gums and inside your lips or cheeks to provide some sugar while awaiting medical help. A doctor will usually give an injection of the hormone glucagon, which quickly raises blood sugar levels.

If you have a fit due to severe lack of glucose, or substantial alcohol consumption or liver disease (in which glucagon does not usually work well), a glucose or dextrose infusion will usually be given instead.

Remember: most people with diabetes have a hypo at some time, and around one in four people with diabetes have one or more severe hypos (requiring help from someone else) every year.

WARNING

If you are taking any medication – tablets or injections – for diabetes, it is important to follow your doctor's instructions carefully on how often to take it. If you want to make changes to your diet, or to start taking vitamin, mineral or herbal supplements, it is important that you discuss these with your doctor first. You must be fully aware of how to monitor your blood glucose levels regularly, and confident in how to adjust your medication if your blood glucose control improves (or worsens).

Lowering your risk

In this chapter, we'll be taking a broad look at the risk factors for diabetes, how to get a handle on your own risk, and basic advice on how to go about reducing it (the rest of the book covers the details). The focus is, inevitably, on type 2 diabetes and metabolic syndrome, which offer far more scope for prevention. But hearteningly, research is now revealing how new mothers may be able to lower the risk of their infants developing type 1 diabetes.

Protecting against type 1 diabetes

It has been found that if mothers breastfeed their babies exclusively for at least the first two months of their lives, the infants are given some protection against type 1 diabetes. A study from Yorkshire, for example, found that exclusive breastfeeding was associated with those offspring being a third less likely to develop type 1 diabetes later in life, compared to similar babies who weren't breastfed.[7] And an Australian study found evidence of an association between type 1 diabetes and exposure to cows' milk in the first months of life; giving it before the baby's third month significantly increased the risk of diabetes, whereas exclusive breastfeeding for three or more months was associated with a protective effect.[8] So it seems fair to say that in a baby's first few months, breastfeeding and holding off exposure to cows' milk may lower the baby's risk of developing type 1 diabetes. In any case, this regime is standard medical advice.

Optimum intakes of some vitamins and minerals also seem to have a protective effect against developing diabetes in epidemiological surveys. Low blood levels of vitamin D, for example, may increase the risk of diabetes, which might explain why diagnosis is less common in summer months, when vitamin D is naturally made in the skin on exposure to sublight. How it protects is unknown, but one study has found that giving a child vitamin D supplements (2000IU daily) can reduce their risk of developing type 1 diabetes by over 80 per cent.[9]

Protecting against metabolic syndrome and type 2 diabetes

Type 2 diabetes may be on the rise, but the good news is that you don't have to join the trend – even if the disease runs in your family. A central message of this book is that you can help to postpone or even prevent the development of metabolic syndrome and type 2 diabetes by taking steps to improve your diet, maintain a healthy weight and exercise regularly.

We've seen how close the link between obesity and type 2 diabetes is, for example: around 75 per cent of people with this form of diabetes are overweight, and it has been estimated that as many as 85 per cent of cases could be prevented by achieving and maintaining an optimal weight. So far, clinical trials have suggested that losing weight, boosting activity levels and improving diet can delay the onset of type 2 diabetes and even reduce your risk of developing it by 58 per cent.

As we saw in Chapter 1, obesity is only part of the story. You'll remember that metabolic syndrome is a combination of high blood pressure, high levels of blood fats and a cluster of other factors, including obesity, that can predispose you to developing type 2 diabetes. So if you have been diagnosed with metabolic syndrome, or if your doctor discovered you have high blood pressure or high levels of triglycerides during a routine checkup, getting these problems under control can lower your chances of sliding into type 2 diabetes.

We'll be looking at the major risk factors one by one, and how to tackle them. Treating metabolic syndrome holistically, with a regime taking into account its characteristic cluster of signs and symptoms, is also discussed in Chapter 13.

Overcoming obesity

Since 1980, the number of obese people has trebled in the West, and at least 20 per cent of women and 25 per cent of men there are now obese. Many more are overweight, bringing the overall total of people carrying too much weight to two-thirds of men, and over half of all women. And as we've seen increasingly in the news, obesity in children is also on the rise.

In Chapter 1 we saw how obesity is now recognised as the most important, modifiable, independent risk factor for developing type 2 diabetes. Obesity also doubles the risk of premature death from a number of other serious health problems, including coronary heart disease and stroke, and cuts seven years off your life – whether you're a man, woman, smoker or non-smoker.

The most dangerous weight gain is the apple-shape, 'spare-tyre' or pot-bellied kind, where weight gathers around the waist, because people with this condition are most at risk of developing metabolic syndrome. Variously called visceral, central, truncal or android obesity, it indicates a waist size of more than 94cm in men, and 80cm in women. Once waist size is greater than 102cm for men or 88cm for women, the likelihood of having metabolic syndrome is very high. For Asian men, risk is greatest in those with a waist circumference greater than 90cm, and for Asian women, risks increase significantly above a waist size of 80cm.

Obesity and metabolic syndrome: The inside story

The exact link between obesity and metabolic syndrome is not yet fully understood. The most plausible theory is that high circulating levels of free fatty acids (FFAs) found in people who are overweight interfere with their glucose metabolism. If your FFA levels are raised, muscle cells can burn them as an alternative fuel source, and will take up and use less glucose.

This in turn may cause your blood glucose levels to rise. High FFA levels also tend to promote the production of new glucose in your liver, which will then enter your circulation and may then raise blood sugar levels further if cells cannot absorb and use it properly.

Another theory is that when fat stores are full, they give out a signal to try to reduce the amount of glucose that enters these cells. This produces insulin resistance. The signal has not yet been identified, but a number of substances produced by fat stores are possible candidates, including a hormone that has been named 'resistin'. Two other fat cell hormones, adiponectin and leptin, may also be involved.

Recent research also suggests that obesity is linked with widespread inflammation throughout the body. Coronary heart disease is also associated with inflammation, which provides a possible causative connection between these two conditions.

Measuring overweight and obesity There are a number of ways of measuring overweight and obesity. The body mass index, for instance, is a fairly reliable way of measuring the total amount of fat you're carrying – as opposed to just weight. If you're overweight or think you might be obese, it's important to measure your BMI: people with significant obesity (that is, a BMI greater than 35kg/m^2) are 40 times more likely to develop diabetes than people of normal weight.

Body mass index

Called the body mass index (BMI) or Quetelet's index, this will help give an accurate picture of your body fat stores. You obtain the BMI by dividing your weight (in kilograms) by the square of your height (in metres):

$$\text{BMI} = \frac{\text{weight (kg)}}{\text{height} \times \text{height (m}^2)}$$

When you've calculated your BMI, you can use the following table –

based on the 1998 World Health Organization guidelines – to interpret the results:

BMI	weight band
≤18.5	Underweight
18.5 – 24.9	Healthy range
25 – 29.9	Overweight
30 – 39.9	Obese
≥ 40	Extremely obese

Let's say your height is 1.7m (5ft 7in), and your weight 76kg (12 stone). Your BMI is calculated as 76 divided by 1.7 x 1.7 = 26.3kg/m^2 – which means you are slightly overweight.

As you can see from the chart above, a BMI of 30kg/m^2 classes a person as obese. This calculation is occasionally misleading. For example, bodybuilders with excessive muscle mass may have a BMI of up to this figure, yet not actually be overweight or obese. Also, for people aged 60 or more, a slightly raised BMI of up to 27 is acceptable, as it doesn't seem to reduce life expectancy.

Although it's not as accurate an indicator of obesity, a chart showing the healthy weight range for your height ratio can also be helpful.

Height		Optimum healthy weight range	
metres	feet	kg	stones
1.47	4'10"	40.0 – 53.8	6st 4 – 8st 7
1.50	4'11"	41.6 – 56.0	6st 8 – 8st 11
1.52	5ft	42.7 – 57.5	6st 10 – 9st 1
1.55	5'1"	44.5 – 59.8	7st – 9st 7
1.57	5'2"	45.6 – 61.4	7st 2 – 9st 9
1.60	5'3"	47.4 – 63.8	7st 6 – 10st
1.63	5'4"	49.2 – 66.2	7st 10 – 10st 6
1.65	5'5"	50.4 – 67.8	7st 13 – 10st 9
1.68	5'6"	52.2 – 70.3	8st 3 – 11st
1.70	5'7"	53.5 – 72.0	8st 6 – 11st 4
1.73	5'8"	55.4 – 74.5	8st 10 – 11st 10

continued overleaf

Height		Optimum healthy weight range	
1.75	5'9"	56.7 – 76.3	8st 13 – 11st 13
1.78	5'10"	58.6 – 78.9	9st 3 – 12st 6
1.80	5'11"	59.9 – 80.7	9st 6 – 12st 10
1.83	6 ft	62.0 – 83.4	9st 11 – 13st 1
1.85	6'1"	63.3 – 85.2	9st 13 – 13st 5
1.88	6'2"	65.4 – 88.0	10st 4 – 13st 12
1.90	6'3"	66.8 – 89.9	10st 7 – 14st 2
1.93	6'4"	68.9 – 92.8	10st 11 – 14st 8

Based on a BMI range of 18.5 – 24.9kg/m^2 with figures rounded upwards

Losing the excess weight Weight loss is now an industry, and if you've grappled with it in your life you'll have encountered the huge range of 'sure-fire' methods for shedding excess pounds.

But the best way to vanquish obesity permanently is to switch to a better way of eating without feeling you're actually on a diet. Look on it as a healthy eating plan for the rest of your life, rather than a temporary slimming phase. If you're overweight and concerned about developing metabolic syndrome or type 2 diabetes, or if you are already living with these conditions, Chapters 5 and 6 offer easy-to-follow, sensible dietary advice designed especially for you. You'll find up-to-date information on weight loss, comparing how the classic low-fat/high-fibre approach and the very low-calorie diets (VLCDs) weigh up next to the increasingly popular low-carbohydrate, higher-protein way of eating advocated by the late Dr Atkins.

It has also been found that exercise alone can help to prevent diabetes, so combining your new healthy diet with the right exercise plan can be doubly protective against the condition. But how much do you need to do to cut risk effectively? Different trials have come up with different results.

In half of adults at risk of developing diabetes, an effective level of moderate-intensity exercise (such as brisk walking) varied from 30 minutes a day to 150 minutes a week. It has been found that both aerobic and resistance training boost insulin sensitivity – and thus glucose uptake in cells. In fact, one bout of exercise can increase insulin sensitivity for at least 16 hours! Note, too, that regularly exercised muscles are more insulin-sensitive. (See

Appendix 1 for a full discussion of the research on exercise and diabetes.)

It is therefore important to try to build at least 30 minutes of exercise into your daily timetable. This 30 minutes doesn't even have to be taken all at once – you could break it up into three bouts of 10 minutes, as long as it is moderate exercise – enough to make you feel slightly breathless. To tell if you are exercising at the right level, take the Talk Test: if you can't talk while exercising, you are over-exerting yourself.

Tips on how to increase your activity levels painlessly

- Walk or run up stairs rather than taking the lift or escalator
- Choose one evening a week when you don't watch TV – go to the gym, kick a ball around or go cycling/swimming with family or friends
- Take up an active hobby such as ballroom dancing, bowls, swimming, golf, rambling, cycling or horseriding and make new friends
- Dig out an old skipping rope, trampoline or other exercise equipment you already have that's just sitting there gathering dust. Use it while watching the evening news
- Walk or cycle reasonable distances rather than taking the car
- Cycle or walk to a local park or a country pub at the weekend
- When staying at home, put more effort into DIY, cleaning and gardening
- Reinstate the old tradition of a family walk after Sunday lunch – kick leaves, skim stones, throw a frisbee – have fun!

If you have a choice, try to exercise during the morning, as this means your metabolism burns faster for the rest of the day and may help you lose more weight overall. Recent evidence is also suggesting that some drugs can help some obese people lose weight, and significantly lower their risk of developing type 2 diabetes. See Appendix 2 on page 245 for a discussion of these.

Added benefits of weight loss If, after adopting your new, active, nutritionally sound lifestyle, you lose just 10kg in weight, you'll see a number of beneficial knock-on effects: you will lower your blood pressure by an average of 10/20mmHg, reduce your triglycerides by 30 per cent, and cut your harmful LDL cholesterol levels by 15 per cent while increasing your good HDL cholesterol by at least 8 per cent. In other words, you will be dismantling or preventing metabolic syndrome – as well as reducing your overall risk of premature death by 20 per cent and your risk of a diabetes-related death by as much as 30 per cent. On top of that, your quality of life will also improve – you'll experience less back and joint pain, less breathlessness, a boost in fertility and a better night's sleep.

Now let's look in more detail at those other, linked risk factors.

Lowering high blood pressure

Blood pressure (BP) is necessary: it keeps your blood circulating. When it's normal, your BP varies naturally throughout the day and goes up and down in response to your emotions and level of activity. If you have high blood pressure, or hypertension, however, your BP remains consistently raised, even at rest.

Hypertension is often referred to as the 'silent killer' because, even when your blood pressure is dangerously high, you can feel relatively well. It can also make you feel dizzy, under the weather, or suffer pounding headaches – but most people feel nothing at all.

Overall, it is estimated that in the UK, more than 1 in 3 adults (37 per cent of men, and 34 per cent of women) have hypertension – a total of 16 million people. As many as 2 out of 3 people with diabetes will develop it, so if you know you have metabolic syndrome or diabetes, keeping track of your blood pressure is probably second nature. But if you don't, and you haven't had your BP checked in the last few years, book an appointment now – especially if high blood pressure, diabetes or heart problems run in your family.

Measuring your blood pressure Blood pressure (BP) is measured according to the length of a column of mercury it can support, so the units used are 'millimetres of mercury', or mmHg. Blood pressure readings are given as a higher figure over a lower figure, such as 120/80mmHg. The higher figure is the pressure in your circulation when your heart contracts to pump blood around your body. The lower figure is the pressure in your system between beats when your heart is at rest.

Your doctor will measure your blood pressure during a normal checkup. Chemists also sell blood pressure monitors for home use, and some pharmacists will even check your blood pressure for you as part of their service

If you have high blood pressure and monitor your BP at home with a wrist monitor, be aware that an accurate reading is only obtained after you have been sitting quietly for a few minutes, with your wrist held at the same level as the heart. You should also keep your body – and especially your arm – still while the blood pressure measurement is made. New technology has now made an accurate measurement easier.

Assessing your risk   The British Hypertension Society recently announced new guidelines on how doctors should treat high blood pressure, as it is also important to focus on other heart disease risk factors including raised cholesterol levels and the risk of blood clots. They recommend that adults should have their blood pressure checked at least every five years until the age of 80. Those with 'high normal' levels of 130/85 to 139/89mmHg, and those who have had high readings at any time, should have their BP checked annually. The average of two readings at each of a number of visits should be used when deciding whether or not to treat. Drug treatment is recommended when blood pressure is consistently 160/100mmHg or higher, while those with a BP of 140/90 to 159/99mmHg should be offered treatment if they have a complication such as diabetes or metabolic syndrome that increases their risk of heart or circulatory problems.

If you have diabetes, your doctor will usually aim to reduce your blood pressure to less than 130/80mmHg if your kidney function is normal, or to less than 125/75mmHg if there is more than 1g protein per 24 hours in your urine. More than one antihypertensive drug is usually needed to achieve these targets.

The new treatment guidelines also suggest which drugs doctors should use, based on the so-called AB/CD rule. Those who are under 55 years of age and non-black should initially be started on drug groups A (an ACE inhibitor or angiotensin receptor blocker) or B (a beta-blocker), while those who are 55 years or older, or black, should receive drug groups C (calcium channel blocker) or D (a diuretic) at first.

This is because younger people and non-blacks tend to have higher levels of an enzyme, renin, which is inhibited by drug groups A and B, while older and black people tend to have low levels of renin and therefore do not respond as well to these groups of drugs. Most people will require more than one drug, however, and if BP does not improve satisfactorily with this initial approach, A or B may be combined with C or D. The combination of drug groups B (a beta-blocker) and D (a diuretic) is not recommended, however, as one side-effect of this combination is that it might actually increase your risk of developing type 2 diabetes. People in both groups who require three drugs to control their blood pressure will therefore all receive drugs from groups A, D and C.

Lowering high blood pressure is essential because of the massive damage it can do. When blood is forced through your system at high pressure, it damages the lining of important arteries. This can lead to a stroke when blood vessels in the brain are damaged, angina or a heart attack when coronary arteries are damaged, and cardiac failure when the heart finds it difficult to pump blood into a highly pressured bloodstream. It can also damage your sight when blood vessels in the eyes are affected, and cause kidney failure when blood vessels in the kidneys are damaged – especially in people who have diabetes.

So lowered blood pressure, like weight loss if you're obese, boosts health in countless ways. By taking away one of the harmful 'building blocks' of metabolic syndrome, you significantly reduce your chances of developing diabetes.

Causes One of the main causes of high blood pressure is age, which hardens and narrows arteries. 'Lifestyle' causes include overweight and obesity, smoking, drinking too much alcohol, eating too much salt, stress, lack of exercise, and the side effects of some drugs. Some diseases cause it, and it also runs in some families. High blood pressure is also linked with high levels of blood fats including cholesterol and triglycerides, and abnormally raised blood levels of the amino acid homocysteine, which can damage blood vessel linings (see page 152).

Getting blood pressure under control If you are diagnosed with hypertension, you need to get the necessary changes in diet and lifestyle in place as soon as possible. The benefits will be tremendous.

Your doctor may also prescribe antihypertensive medication. Six classes of drug are available to lower high blood pressure, and depending on the severity of your hypertension, your doctor may prescribe a number of them, or just one.

The 20-year UK Prospective Diabetes Study investigated treatments to improve management and prevent complications in over 5000 people newly diagnosed with type 2 diabetes. Results showed that tight control of high blood pressure significantly reduced the risk of any diabetes-related complications by almost a quarter (24 per cent), diabetes-related deaths by 32 per cent, stroke by 44 per cent and heart failure by 56 per cent. The 1998 Hypertension Optimal Treatment (HOT) study found that people with diabetes who achieved a target diastolic blood pressure of 81.1mmHg showed a 51 per cent reduction in heart attack and stroke and a 60 per cent reduction in deaths from these major cardiovascular events.

So what do you need to do to lower your blood pressure significantly? Here are the key steps (and note that more detailed information on much of the following can be found in Chapters 5 and 6):

• If you smoke, try to stop. Chemicals in cigarettes can damage artery linings, and raise your BP. Within 20 minutes of stopping

61

smoking, your blood pressure and pulse rate will fall significantly. Within eight hours, levels of carbon monoxide in your blood will drop to normal and oxygen levels in your blood will rise. Within 48 hours, your blood will thin enough to reduce your risk of a heart attack or stroke. And within three months the blood supply to your limbs, hands and feet will have increased.

- Get active. Try to walk as much as possible, and use the stairs instead of the lift. Aim to exercise for at least 30 minutes, five times a week and preferably every day. Exercise tones up your heart and circulation, improves the strength and efficiency of your heart's pumping action, and helps you maintain a healthy weight. Note that exercise does not usually cause hypoglycaemia in people with type 2 diabetes, so extra carbohydrate is generally unnecessary. People with type 1 diabetes should not start an exercise programme without first seeking medical advice about how to adjust their insulin regime and carbohydrate intake.

- Lose excess weight. This can sometimes lower your BP enough to reduce any need for drug treatment.

- Give up heavy drinking. Not everyone realises that excess alcohol can affect your heart and circulation as well as your liver. Limit yourself to a maximum of two or three units of alcohol per day – and have regular alcohol-free days, too.

- De-stress. Try to avoid stressful situations, and take time out to relax and overcome the effects of stress hormones. Meditation may well be worth trying. A study published in *Hypertension* (the journal of the American Heart Association) showed that Transcendental Meditation could reduce systolic BP by an average of 11mmHg and diastolic BP by 6mmHg within three months. As well as reducing stress, TM lowers anxiety and raised serum cholesterol, and improves your quality of sleep as well as helping you to stop smoking, lower your alcohol consumption and get off recreational drugs.

- Up your intake of fruit and vegetables. Aim to eat at least five to eight or nine servings of fruit and veg a day.

- Cut back on salt. Don't add it during cooking or at the table. Doing this could lower blood pressure by at least 5mmHg. There is now a general consensus that salt intake should be reduced to less than 6g per day for adults, but on average we consume

10 to 12g daily. It has been calculated that reducing salt to less than 6g per day would prevent 60,000 heart attacks and strokes a year in the UK, 50 per cent of them fatal. Where salt is essential, use mineral-rich rock salt rather than table salt, or sparingly use a potassium-rich, low-sodium brand of salt. In one study, those taking antihypertensive medication were able to halve their dose under medical supervision, simply by increasing the potassium content of their food.

- Consume healthy fats in sensible quantities. Rapeseed, olive, flaxseed, fish and walnuts oils all have beneficial effects on cholesterol levels.
- Drink either green, 'white' or black tea. Tea has beneficial effects on circulation due to the powerful antioxidants they contain. Those drinking at least four cups of tea a day are half as likely to have a heart attack as non-tea drinkers and less likely to suffer from high blood pressure.
- Consider taking magnesium, garlic and co-enzyme Q10, all of which may help to lower a high BP.

Lowering blood fat

As we've seen, the fats in your blood are mainly made up of cholesterol and triglycerides. In essence, cholesterol is a fatty substance needed for making cell membranes and hormones, and it can be beneficial or harmful, depending on type.

There are two main sources – the kind made in your liver from dietary saturated fats (around 800mg per day) and the kind you get pre-formed in your diet (around 300mg per day). Circulating low density lipoprotein (LDL) cholesterol and very low density lipoprotein (VLDL) cholesterol are the 'bad' cholesterols, as they are linked with hardening and furring up of artery walls, high blood pressure and coronary heart disease. High density lipoprotein (HDL) cholesterol is often referred to as 'good' cholesterol, as it protects against heart disease by transporting LDL and VLDL cholesterol away from the arteries and back to the liver for processing.

If you have metabolic syndrome, you'll have a higher level of bad cholesterol and a lower level of good cholesterol. Usually, you will have raised total and VLDL cholesterol, raised triglycerides, reduced levels of the beneficial HDL cholesterol and relatively normal levels of LDL cholesterol. Although the level of LDL cholesterol may not have changed, the balance of LDL cholesterol particles probably has. So there will be more small, dense fat particles, which are more strongly linked with hardening and furring up of the arteries, and less of the larger, fluffier and less harmful LDL particles.

Measuring blood fat levels If you have diabetes or metabolic syndrome, you need to watch your levels of blood fats. They should be checked at least annually. Levels for people with diabetes, as suggested by the International Task Force for Prevention of Coronary Heart Disease, are as follows:

Safe Levels of Blood Fats for People with Diabetes

Type of fat	No evidence of arterial disease	Evidence of arterial disease
LDL cholesterol	<3.4mmol/l	<2.6mmol/l
HDL cholesterol	>0.9mmol/l	>0.9mmol/l
Triglycerides	<1.8mmol/l	<1.8mmol/l

In people with type 2 diabetes, blood triglyceride levels and reduced levels of beneficial HDL cholesterol are more strongly associated with coronary heart disease than total and LDL cholesterol.

Getting blood fats under control For many people, diet and lifestyle changes alone can lower their cholesterol levels. Eating well and exercising sensibly are important, and, starting with Chapter 7, you will find many nutritional and herbal supplements that treat high cholesterol levels directly.

Often, however, genetic factors can make it difficult to lower cholesterol and triglyceride levels through diet and exercise alone, unless you are prepared to make a dramatic change such as following the low-carbohydrate nutritional approach advocated by the late Dr Atkins (see Chapter 6) or a similar low glycaemic diet. Low-fat diets alone are not normally enough, as they still provide the excess carbohydrates from which your body makes glucose and triglyceride fats. So if you have high levels of blood fats, you might need drug treatments to reduce the risk of premature death, especially if you have other risk factors for heart disease – for instance, if you are diabetic, smoke, are overweight and/or have high blood pressure.

Until recently, prescription medicines available to lower blood cholesterol levels targeted its production in the liver. These include the statins (including atorvastin, fluvastatin, pravastatin, simvastatin, rosuvastatin), bile acid sequestrants (such as cholestyramine, colestipol) and the fibrates (bezafibrate, ciprofibrate, fenofibrate, gemfibrozil). Unfortunately, these drugs are not without side effects, and are also responsible for blocking the production of an important substance, co-enzyme Q10, in the body (see page 136). If you and your doctor decide that a statin is right for you, then it is a good idea to take CoQ10 supplements to ensure you have enough for the healthy working of your muscles – especially the heart.

Recently, a new class of drug for lowering cholesterol levels was developed. Known as a cholesterol absorption inhibitor, ezetimibe works by blocking the absorption of cholesterol from the intestines. Cholesterol absorption inhibitors are designed to be taken together with a statin, so both production of cholesterol in the liver and its absorption from the intestines is reduced.

The multi-treatment approach to metabolic syndrome

So far we've looked at the conditions making up metabolic syndrome – which are also risk factors for developing type 2 diabetes – one by one. And the medical treatment of metabolic syndrome has in fact tended to focus on single risk factors such as high blood pressure, obesity and abnormally high blood fat levels. But as it's a cluster of conditions, multi-tier treatment is a sensible approach. In fact, it is now known that simultaneously treating multiple risk factors is very effective for the most severely affected people.

First off, you need to follow my suggestions for exercise, outlined above, and a suitable, low-glycaemic index diet (page 70).

Treatment may involve taking low doses of aspirin (to reduce blood clotting) and a statin (to reduce cholesterol levels even if not dramatically raised), plus setting up stricter targets for controlling blood pressure and impaired glucose tolerance. This combined approach can reduce the risk of a heart attack or stroke by at least 50 per cent. One class of oral hypoglycaemic drugs, the glitazones (see page 46) is particularly helpful, as it not only lowers glucose levels, but also has beneficial effects on blood pressure, blood fat levels and inflammation. Treatment with an anti-obesity drug (such as orlistat or sibutramine) is also helpful in reducing apple-shape obesity; see Appendix 2 for a full discussion of these drugs, including recent research on them.

5

Healthy eating: The basics

If you've just been diagnosed with diabetes or metabolic syndrome, you could be thinking that as far as food is concerned, the good times are over. Now, you imagine, you face a grossly restricted, deadly dull 'diabetic' diet for the rest of your life.

Not so. Special 'diabetic' diets are no more. Instead, you simply need to follow the same healthy eating guidelines recommended for everyone. That means a diet that is high in fibre and low in processed fats, supplies at least five servings of fruit and vegetables a day and avoids excess sugar, refined carbohydrates, alcohol and salt. The focus should be on fresh wholefoods, as minimally processed as possible, and away from ready meals and the rest of the highly processed packaged foods that cram today's supermarket shelves, and are laden with salt, trans fats, sugar and preservatives. People with metabolic syndrome or type 2 diabetes may do even better on a low-carbohydrate, higher-protein diet, as there is mounting evidence to show how well it balances blood sugar.

The traditional approach to healthy eating

Broadly speaking, the traditional recommended healthy diet divides up your daily energy needs, as calories, like this:
- 50 per cent to 55 per cent as carbohydrates – mainly starchy carbohydrates such as baked potatoes or brown rice, rather than refined, processed carbohydrates such as white flour and sugar

- 30 to 35 per cent as fat
- 10 to 15 per cent as protein.

It is important not to skip meals, as hunger can lead you down the quick-fix route to grabbing refined carbohydrates (a scone, a pastry, a biscuit) for fast energy, 'just this once'. And that, of course, spells disaster whatever form of diabetes or pre-diabetic condition you have. Eating regular meals that include a wide variety of foods and are high in fibre will help keep your blood sugar balanced. Those five servings of fruit or vegetables per day will give you abundant vitamins and other micronutrients, as well as important dietary fibre. And finally, you need to stay hydrated, so drink 2 to 3 litres of water (which can include tea and herbal teas) every day.

A low-GI diet will include so-called 'slow' carbs that are processed relatively slowly in the body. As a result of this, they produce less dramatic swings in blood glucose. A typical day's menu on the low-GI diet might look something like this:

Breakfast
Porridge, Weetabix or other relatively unprocessed, sugar-free cereal with chopped apple and semi-skimmed milk, OR
Two slices wholemeal or rye toast with a poached or boiled egg and an apple, pear or handful of berries, OR
Low-sugar or homemade baked beans on wholemeal or rye toast.
Cup of tea with a dash of semi-skimmed milk.

Lunch
Baked potato filled with tuna, low-sugar baked beans or chicken salad, with a mixed salad or green vegetables, OR
Sardines in olive oil or a kipper with rye bread or oatcakes and salad, OR
A sandwich made with wholemeal bread or brown pitta and chicken, turkey, cottage cheese or tuna, with a mixed salad.
Apple, pear or handful of berries,
Cup of herbal tea.

Dinner
Piece of lean meat (chicken, turkey or game), tofu steak or fish,

AND
multicoloured vegetables (spinach, carrots, red peppers, celery, tomatoes and the like), stir-fried or in a salad,
Apple, pear or handful of berries,
Cup of tea.

In contrast, a controlled carbohydrate plan such as the Atkins nutritional approach limits intakes of carbohydrates more strictly, and a typical day's eating when following the early phases of a controlled carbohydrate plan might look like this:

Breakfast
Two-egg omelette with cheese and mushrooms,
Two rashers of bacon, rocket salad,
Bowl of fresh berries (blueberries, raspberries, strawberries),
Cafetière coffee made with cream.

Lunch
Grilled salmon steak served with a large mixed leaf salad, parmesan cheese and Caesar salad dressing,
Platter of cheese with grapes and walnuts (NB no biscuits or bread),
Cup of herbal tea.

Dinner
Grilled beef steak with garlic and herb butter AND multicoloured vegetables (spinach, carrots, red peppers, celery, tomatoes and the like), stir-fried or in a salad,
Chocolate mousse made with artificial sweetener,
Cup of tea.

As you progress through the Atkins nutritional approach, you will introduce more carbohydrates from sources such as vegetables, low-glycaemic fruits, aged cheeses, nuts, seeds and wholegrains until you reach your goal weight. Eventually you may be able to eat as much as 120g of net carbohydrates per day or more, and can include small amounts of carbohydrate-rich foods such as potatoes, rice, pasta and even bread in your diet.

Olive, walnut or other kinds of recommended oils (see page 79) can be used in salad dressings when following either eating plan.

Now we'll look in detail at the most important aspects of healthy eating from the diabetic perspective. That means finding out which foods balance blood glucose, and which don't; as well as which foods reduce the risk of coronary heart disease and circulatory problems, and which don't. So I've concentrated on carbohydrates, proteins, fats, and the crucial antioxidants found in fruits, vegetables and other sources.

All about carbohydrates

Keeping your glucose in balance is your top health priority. And as carbohydrates are the main source of glucose, you need to be sure you're getting the kind that will make this task easiest. Refined carbohydrates such as white sugar found in cakes and sweets contain simple sugars such as glucose, which quickly raise blood sugar levels. You need to avoid these. Unrefined carbohydrates such as starches found in oats, or wholewheat spaghetti are made up of chains of simple sugars, which must first be broken down into more basic units before they affect blood glucose levels. These 'slow-releasing' carbohydrates are generally better for you.

People with type 1 diabetes may be encouraged by their health-carers to count the grams of carbohydrate they eat during the day as this helps them eat a wider range of foods by combining those with a higher carb count with those of a lower carb count. This can help you control your blood glucose levels more closely and is relatively easy as food labels will include carbohydrate content. Books that include carbohydrate counts are widely available (eg see bibliography). If your doctor wishes you to count carbohydrates, they will provide detailed information to help you do this.

The glycaemic index

Back in 1981, researchers invented a way to determine precisely how a food affects blood glucose levels. This is the glycaemic index (GI) – a chart that compares each carbohydrate food to pure glucose in terms of how fast they break down into glucose in the body. Glucose is given a standard glycaemic index of 100, and other carbohydrates are given a value relative to this. Parsnips have a very high GI, at 97, while fructose (a sugar found in fruit, vegetables and honey) has a low GI of 23.

Glycaemic Index

FOOD	GI	FOOD	GI
Glucose	100	Kiwi fruit	52
Parsnips	97	Bran cereal	51
Carrots	95	Crisps	51
Baked potatoes	85	Strawberry jam	51
Cornflakes	81	Cake	50
Doughnuts	76	Chocolate bar	49
Weetabix	75	Peas	47
White bread	73	Grapes	46
Wholemeal bread	72	Baked beans	44
Potatoes, mashed	70	White spaghetti, boiled	44
Shredded Wheat	67	Orange	42
Raisins	64	Wholemeal spaghetti, boiled	37
White basmati rice	64	Apple	38
Honey	62	Pears	38
Chocolate biscuit	59	Tomato soup	38
New potatoes, boiled	59	Ice cream	36
Apricots	57	Whole milk	30
Banana	56		
Potato chips	56	Very low GI foods (less than 30)	
Sweetcorn	56	Butter, cheese, eggs, fish, grapefruit,
Brown rice	55	green vegetables, meat, nuts,
Mango	55	plums, seafood, pulses (soy beans,
Porridge oats	54	kidney beans and the like)

Note that values differ between different sources. Typical values are given in the above table

In essence, a low GI is below 55; a medium GI is 56 to 69; and a high GI is over 70.

For people with diabetes or metabolic syndrome, the glycaemic index initially seemed like a good idea. Balancing blood sugar was all down to avoiding foods with a high GI and choosing those with a low to moderate GI. It also allowed them to combine foods with a high GI, such as potatoes, with those that have a lower GI, such as beans, to help even out fluctuations in blood glucose levels.

Glycaemic load

However, the GI is not a perfect system. The method used to devise it was to feed volunteers whatever quantity of a food contains 50g of useable carbohydrate. But since carrots, for example, contain only about 7 per cent carbohydrate, eating 50g of carbohydrate from carrots alone means you would have to eat around a pound and a half of them for the test, giving a spuriously high GI value of 95. This is obviously not realistic. Also, the GI is based on eating a single food rather than a mixed meal, as normally occurs. When you eat, say, brown rice with chicken, or fruit with nuts, the amount of fat, fibre and protein you consume with the carbohydrate will have a balancing effect on blood sugar swings.

So a better measure was devised: the glycaemic load (GL). This takes into account the actual amount of food eaten in a typical serving.

You calculate GL in this way:

$$\text{Glycemic load (GL)} = \frac{\text{GI x net carbohydrate content (without fibre)}}{100}$$

So, a low GL is up to 10; a medium GL is 11 to 19; and a high GL is over 20.

Using GL as a measure, carrots have a value of around 6, which is classed as low, as a typical serving will have little significant effect on blood glucose levels. By contrast, white spaghetti, which has a relatively low GI of 44, has a relatively high GL of 18.

The table below shows both glycaemic index and glycaemic load scores for a number of carbohydrates.

**Glycaemic Index and Glycaemic Load Values
for Selected Foods**

Food	Glycaemic Index (glucose=100)	Serving size	Carbohydrate per serving (g)	Glycaemic Load per serving
Potato (baked)	85	1 medium (150g)	30	26
Cornflakes	81	30g	26	21
Doughnut	76	47g	23	17
White bread	73	30g	14	10
Table sugar (sucrose)	68	10g	10	7
White rice (boiled)	64	150g	36	23
Brown rice (boiled)	55	150g	33	18
Spaghetti, white, boiled	44	140g	40	18
Spaghetti, wholewheat, boiled	37	140g	37	14
Oranges, raw	42	120g	11	5
Pears, raw	38	120g	11	4
Apples, raw	38	120g	15	6
All-Bran™ cereal	38	30g	23	9
Skimmed milk	32	250ml	13	4
Lentils, dried, boiled	29	150g	18	5
Kidney beans, dried, boiled	28	150g	25	7
Pearl barley, boiled	25	150g	42	11
Cashew nuts	22	30g	9	2
Peanuts	14	30g	6	1

All about proteins

Dietary proteins are made up of building blocks known as amino acids, which can be linked together to form chains. Chains with 10 to 100 amino acids tend to be called polypeptides, while chains of over 100 amino acids fold into complex three-dimensional shapes known as proteins.

Dietary proteins are digested to release their amino acid – a process that starts with stomach enzymes. Once they have been absorbed into your body, amino acids are used as building blocks to make all the 50,000 different proteins and polypeptides we need to function properly. Some of these proteins play a structural role (such as collagen), some regulate metabolic reactions (enzymes, hormones) while others are vital for immunity (antibodies). The protein in your body is constantly being broken down and reformed under the control of growth hormone – mostly while you are asleep – at a rate of around 80 to 100g a day. Most muscle protein is renewed every 6 months, for example, while 98 per cent of your total body proteins are renewed within 1 year.

A total of 21 amino acids are now known to be important for human health. Of these, 12 – the non-essential amino acids – can be made in the body from other building blocks, but the remaining 9 cannot be synthesised in the amounts needed by your metabolism, and must therefore come from your diet. These are known as the nutritionally essential amino acids.

Essential amino acids

Histidine	Phenylalanine
Isoleucine	Threonine
Leucine	Tryptophan
Lysine	Valine
Methionine	

Non-essential amino acids

Alanine	Proline
Arginine	Serine
Asparagine	Cysteine
Aspartate	Selenocysteine (only recently recognised as
Glutamate	essential for health)
Glutamine	Tyrosine
Glycine	

When your diet is rich in protein, excess amino acids cannot be stored in their original form. Excess protein that is not needed for growth or repair of body tissues must be broken down directly as a fuel for energy, converted into glucose or, if energy is plentiful, converted into glycogen or fatty acids for storage. This is important, because it means that even if you are following a low-glycaemic diet, which provides little dietary glucose, your body can still obtain all the glucose it needs from the proteins in your diet.

Dietary protein can be divided into two groups: first-class proteins, which contain significant quantities of all the essential amino acids (such as meat, fish, eggs and dairy products) and second-class proteins, which contain some essential amino acids but not all (such as vegetables, rice, beans, nuts). Second-class proteins need to be mixed and matched by eating as wide a variety of foods as possible. For instance, the essential amino acid missing from haricot beans is found in bread. So combining cereals with pulses or seeds and nuts provides a balanced amino acid intake. Vegetarians can also obtain a balanced protein intake by eating a combination of five parts rice to one part beans.

The average adult needs to obtain around 56g of protein per day from their food, and most people in the UK obtain significantly more than this.

The lowdown on fats

For many decades now, fat has had a bad press. The truth is that we need fat in our diet. It's an important source of readily available energy, for instance, and we also need to eat it to get the benefits of the important fat-soluble vitamins A, D and E. Vitamin D, for instance, is abundant in oily fish, while seed oils are rich in E.

But there are good fats, and bad fats. So-called 'trans' or hydrogenated fats, found in many processed foods, are emerging as major health risks. By contrast, the essential fatty acids (EFAs) which are found in seeds and oily fish such as salmon are, as their name implies, vital for our health. We'll be looking in more depth at the goodies and baddies among dietary fats below.

Fats: The inside story

Most of the fats we eat are triglycerides. These consist of a molecule of glycerol, made up of three carbon atoms, to which three fatty acids – long chains of hydrogen and carbon atoms – are attached. All together, they look a bit like a capital E. The precise arrangement of atoms within the molecule determines whether triglycerides will be either solid or liquid at room temperature, as well as how they're metabolised in your body. Their structure also determines whether they're saturated, monounsaturated or polyunsaturated. In general, saturated fats tend to be solid at room temperature, while monounsaturated and polyunsaturated fats tend to be oils.

The types of dietary fat

Most dietary fats contain a blend of saturated, monounsaturated and polyunsaturated fats in varying proportions. For example, lard, which most people assume is made up of saturated fat, contains as much as 47 per cent monounsaturated fat. But what do all these terms mean, and what effect do these fats have on our health?

Saturated fats Saturated fats come from animal sources, such as meat and dairy products. Some are converted into cholesterol in the liver, and were traditionally thought of as the baddies when it came to coronary heart disease. But they are now thought to be less important in this respect. In fact, over a third of the saturated fats in milk fat or butter have no effect on blood cholesterol levels – stearic acid, found in milk fat, cocoa butter and meat fat, being a prime example.

One of the longest-running studies into coronary heart disease found no link between high blood cholesterol levels and saturated fat intake. In fact, the analysis of data from the Framingham Heart Study found that, while people's intake of saturated fat increased as a proportion of energy from 16.4 per cent in the period 1966 to 1969, to 17 per cent in the period 1984 to 1988, there were concurrently significant decreases in blood total and LDL cholesterol levels.

That doesn't mean you can eat limitless amounts of sirloin steak and butter, however. A high saturated fat intake can be harmful because like all fats, it has a high calorie content. And if combined with a high intake of carbohydrates, too much saturated fat can lead to obesity and serious complications such as high blood pressure.

Polyunsaturated fats There are two main families of polyunsaturated fats or fatty acids, or PUFAs, in the diet:

- omega-3s, mainly derived from fish oils
- omega-6s, mainly derived from vegetable oils.

These omega fats are known as essential fatty acids or EFAs. And as their name reveals, they are absolutely vital for health. As we can't synthesise all of them in our body, we need to get them from food.

The least complex form of EFA in the omega-3 family is alpha-linolenic acid; in the omega-6 family, it's linoleic acid. These are the two essential fatty acids that we definitely cannot make in our body. Linoleic acid is converted into an EFA called GLA (also found in borage oil and evening primrose oil) in the body, while alpha-linolenic acid or ALA is converted into two EFAs with the unwieldy names of eicosapentaenoic and docosahexaenoic acid, or EPA and DHA. Flaxseeds, pumpkin seeds, green leafy vegetables and walnuts can be an indirect source of EPA and DHA, as they all contain ALA. But the best direct source of EPA and DHA are oily, coldwater fish such as sardines, mackerel and salmon.

Whichever way you get them, this pair are the stars of the fatty acid world. They perform a vital function in our central nervous system, forming part of the fatty portion of our brain as well as the sheaths that protect connections between nerves and keep that brain working smoothly. They also have a thinning effect on your blood, and so help reduce the risk of coronary heart disease and stroke. They help make the membranes of our cells and our arterial walls, as well as prostaglandins, hormone-like substances that help regulate our metabolism. If you have metabolic syndrome or type 2 diabetes, these EFAs provide important protection against damage from insulin resistance, as they calm inflammation in the arteries caused by repeated bursts of glucose in the blood.

The findings on omega-6s present a more problematic picture. Found in sunflower and safflower oils as well as those of borage and evening primrose, they are increasingly linked with inflammatory processes in the body, including coronary heart disease. However, the basic omega-6 fatty acid, linoleic acid, remains *essential*; the real problem is that we tend to consume too much of them in relation to few omega-3s. The ratio of omega-6 to omega-3 in the average Western diet is currently 7:1, but should be something like 3:1, as the imbalance may increase inflammation and the risk of hardening and furring up of the arteries.

This is because, compared with saturated fats, polyunsaturated fats are much more vulnerable to oxidation, a chemical change that can happen when they are heated or exposed to air for any length of time. During oxidation, toxic substances that are believed to harm artery walls are produced. So it's important to take care when using and storing PUFAs. They are best kept in the fridge, and consumed unheated (in salad dressings, for instance, or as supplements). As protection against any oxidation in the body, you should consider taking antioxidant supplements (see page 124).

See below for recommended amounts of PUFAs in the diet. It's very important to ensure you're getting enough, and in the right ratio. If your intake of EFAs is low, your body will use the next best fats available – and that could be saturated fat or even trans fats (see below). This can affect the elasticity and quality of your arteries, for instance.

See Chapter 12 for more on EFAs.

Go fish:
the top source of omega-3s

It's no accident that the healthiest people in the world eat a lot of fish. Italians, Greeks and other Mediterranean peoples, as well as Inuits from the far north, all have some of the lowest levels of coronary heart disease – and are all inveterate fish eaters. What's the connection? Oily fish such as salmon, trout, mackerel and sardines contain the essential omega-3s EPA and DHA, which do the heart huge favours by reducing the stickiness of the blood and platelet clumping, as well as the formation of harmful blood clots and the development of dangerous heart rhythms.

Eating oily fish two or three times a week has been shown to reduce the risk of heart attack and stroke. In fact, eating oily fish at least twice a week can lower your risk of coronary heart disease more effectively than following a low-fat, high-fibre diet. Research also shows that the protective effects of oily fish are seen after only six months and, after two years, those on a high-fish diet are almost a third less likely to die from coronary heart disease than people who don't eat much fish.

Unfortunately, we cannot eat as much fish as might be desirable due to the possible presence of pollutants such as heavy metals, dioxins and polychlorinated biphenyls (PCBs). One option is to take omega-3 fish oil supplements that have been screened for levels of pollutants (see page 224).

The UK's Food Standards Agency recently issued the following advice on oily fish:

> Men and boys, and women past childbearing age or who are not able or intending to have children, can eat up to four portions of oily fish a week before the possible risks might start to outweigh the known health benefits.
>
> Girls and women who may become pregnant at some point in their lives can eat between one and two portions of oily fish a week to get the known health benefits whilst limiting any possible effects on any children that they may have in the future.

Pregnant and breastfeeding women can also eat between one and two portions of oily fish a week, and should do so not just for the health benefits to them but because oily fish also helps the neurological development of their babies. The Agency already advises pregnant women and women intending to become pregnant to avoid shark, marlin and swordfish, and not to eat large amounts of tuna. The reason is that large carnivorous fish come very high up the marine foodchain, and so will have eaten accumulations of mercury from quite a lot of fish.

Occasionally eating more than the amounts of oily fish advised by the FSA isn't harmful.

Monounsaturated fats Like the omega-3s, monounsaturated fats are highly beneficial for health. Found in olive oil, rapeseed oil, walnuts and avocados, the monounsaturated fats are metabolised in such a way that they lower harmful LDL cholesterol levels with no effect on beneficial HDL levels. Because monounsaturates reduce your risk of atherosclerosis, high blood pressure, coronary heart disease and stroke, they are invaluable for people with diabetes. And replacing omega-6s with monounsaturates will have the dual benefit of reducing your risk of coronary heart disease and bringing your dietary ratio of omega-3s and omega-6s into a better balance.

Southern star: olive oil

The Greeks, Spanish and Italians know a thing or two: olive oil is one of the healthiest dietary oils, rich in beneficial monounsaturated oleic acid. If you have metabolic syndrome or type 2 diabetes, oleic acid is all good news because it helps regulate insulin and cholesterol levels, as well as blood pressure.

In one study, when 11 people with type 2 diabetes switched from their usual diet to one rich in olive oil for two months, they experienced a small but significant decrease in fasting glucose and insulin levels. Insulin-stimulated transport of glucose was significantly greater, and dilation in their blood vessels also improved. The researchers concluded that changing from a polyunsaturated to a more monounsaturated diet can reduce insulin resistance in type 2 diabetes, as well as have beneficial effects on the circulation.

Olive oil also reduces the absorption of cholesterol, and is processed in the body to lower harmful LDL cholesterol without modifying desirable HDL cholesterol. And it reduces abnormal blood clotting tendencies. If you use olive oil frequently – in salad dressings and for cooking – you can reduce your risk of developing coronary heart disease by 25 per cent. Several studies which have looked at people recovering from a heart attack have shown that those following a Mediterranean-style diet (rich in olive oil as well as nuts, seeds, fruits and vegetables, and low in red meat) were from 50 to 70 per cent less likely to have another heart attack, or to die from heart problems, than those following their normal diet.

Olive oil is also hugely beneficial for people with high blood pressure. Another study showed that using 30 to 40g olive oil for cooking every day can reduce the need for antihypertensive drugs in people with high blood pressure by almost 50 per cent over a six-month period, compared with only 4 per cent for those randomised to use sunflower oil. All those on the sunflower oil diet continued to need their anti-hypertensive drug treatment, while 80 per cent of the people using olive oil were able to discontinue their drug treatment altogether – a pretty astounding figure.

Note that pure olive oil remains stable at elevated temperatures due to its high levels of monounsaturated fatty acids and the natural antioxidant, vitamin E. Refined olive oil can therefore be heated up to 210°C before chemical changes take place. Virgin and extra virgin olive oils are less stable, however, due to their higher content of heat-sensitive components that contribute to their colour and flavour. Because of this, the smell or taste of virgin olive oil may change if heated above 180°C.

So sauté with pure olive oil and keep virgin or extra virgin olive oils for steaming, braising and dressings. Discard any that begin to smoke or smell odd during use. Ideally, cooking oils should not be reused.

Plant sterols and stanols Plant sterols and stanols are substances with a chemical structure similar to that of animal cholesterol, which are found in virtually all plants. They've been found to have a remarkable effect on levels of harmful cholesterol in the blood, as they interact with the absorption of cholesterol from food. Consuming 2g plant sterols or stanols per day can significantly lower levels of harmful LDL cholesterol and help to protect against heart disease.

A number of foods have now been developed that are fortified with these cholesterol-lowering substances, including spreads and yoghurts such as Benecol and Flora pro-activ. When included in a healthy diet, they help to lower LDL cholesterol by up to 15 per cent within as little as three weeks. Consuming 20 to 25g of a spread containing plant sterols daily can lower LDL cholesterol by 10 to 15 per cent.

Trans fats So far, we've looked in the main at fats that do us good. But inadvertently, many of us in the West are eating a kind of fat that is really harmful: the so-called trans fat. It lurks in all sorts of processed foods, from bakery products and solid cooking fats to some kinds of margarine.

A trans fat is a polyunsaturated oil that has been partially hydrogenated (via the introduction of hydrogen atoms), which has the effect of solidifying it. Some have a 'kinky' structure, in which part of the chain is twisted around on itself. As a result, when trans fats are incorporated into cell membranes, they thicken them and make them more rigid, as the kinks can't be straightened out in the same way as non-trans fatty acids. Artificial trans fats also seem to raise blood levels of LDL cholesterol while lowering HDL cholesterol. So trans fats have been linked with an increased risk of high blood pressure and coronary heart disease. They may also interfere with the way your body handles EFAs so their beneficial effects are not fully realised.

On average in the West, we eat around 5 to 7g of trans fats a day. People who eat a lot of cheap margarine, store-bought cakes, cereals, crisps, biscuits and fried foods end up consuming as much as 25 to 30g of them a day. Concern about their safety has prompted some manufacturers to reformulate margarines and low-fat spreads to reduce their trans-fat content. Some countries have also introduced guidelines aimed at reducing amounts consumed to no more than 2 per cent of people's total energy intake.

Not all trans fats are manufactured. Natural kinds are also produced in the rumen (first stomach) of cattle, sheep and goats. As a result, milk, cheese, butter and meat contain small amounts of trans fats – about 2 to 4 per cent. These naturally occurring trans fats are structurally different from those produced commercially, however, and they have not been implicated in increasing the risk of developing coronary heart disease. This has turned the butter vs margarine controversy on its head, leading some scientists to believe that it is healthier to eat butter than margarine or low-fat spreads.

So should you eat butter rather than margarine? This kind of judgement is a bit of a minefield. The simplest advice is to eat as wide a variety of foods as possible, including a little of everything (butter *and* margarine, if you wish), and to eat nothing to excess. And aim to keep your intake of artificial trans fats from processed foods to the bare minimum.

How much fat should you eat?

Current advice is that no more than 30 to 35 per cent of your daily energy intake should be made up of dietary fats. In real terms, if you're a woman with an average energy intake of 1928 kcal per day, 30 per cent of your food energy intake would amount to around 66g of fat. A tablespoon of dietary fat contains around 15g of fat, so that's a bit more than 4 tablespoons of the kinds of fats I recommend above – olive, nut or seed oils, for instance. (Higher-fat diets may be acceptable, but only in combination with a low-carbohydrate intake, as you'll see in Chapter 6.)

But what proportions of these beneficial fats should you eat? Below you'll find the latest recommendations from the government. (Note, however, that they are based on current advice to eat a low-fat diet, so they don't necessarily reflect the views of those who, like myself, are converted to the benefits of lower-carbohydrate nutritional approaches.)

- Monounsaturated fatty acids (olive or rapeseed oil, avocados) –12 per cent
- Polyunsaturated fatty acids (fish, walnut, pumpkin seed, flaxseed and vegetable oils) – 6 per cent, up to a maximum of 10 per cent, of which linoleic acid should make a minimum of 1 per cent, and linolenic acid a minimum of 0.2 per cent
- Trans fatty acids – 2 per cent
- Saturated fats – 10 per cent (although when eaten as part of a low-carbohydrate diet, intakes of 20 per cent saturated fat has been shown not to affect risk factors for coronary heart disease).

Along with a concentration on olive oil, fish oils and the like, you can further reduce your risk of atherosclerosis, coronary heart disease and stroke in a number of ways: eating foods fortified with plant sterols/stanols, remembering to reduce your intake of omega-6 fatty acids (mainly found in vegetable oils such as soy, corn, safflower and sunflower oils), limiting processed foods in your diet so you can avoid consuming too many trans fats, and increasing the amount of antioxidants – found in fruit, vegetables and supplements – to keep any risks from oxidised oils to a minimum.

Antioxidants: safeguarding health

We've seen how important eating the right carbohydrates, proteins and fats is to keep you in the very best of balanced health. But there are other elements in the picture: antioxidants, for one, which play a crucial role in diabetic health.

Why are antioxidants so important? If you have diabetes, you are particularly vulnerable to abnormal metabolic reactions that result from harmful oxidation reactions involving glucose and so-called 'free radicals'. A free radical is a molecular fragment that is highly unstable, and so able to oxidise other molecules and cell structures in your body when they collide with them. Because of this vulnerability, you'll generally need more antioxidants – including the vitamins A, C and E, and other plant chemicals such as carotenoids and flavonoids – than other people.

Now let's take a swift look at some of the dietary sources of these vital safeguards to health.

Fruit and vegetables

Eating five to nine helpings of fruit and vegetables every day is essential for health. For instance, it's been found that people who eat the most raw and fresh fruit have the lowest risk of developing coronary heart disease and stroke. Fruit, vegetables, seeds and pulses are fabulously rich sources of vitamins (including antioxidants), minerals, fibre and at least 20 non-nutrient substances, known as phytochemicals, that have a beneficial effect on health. Some of these substances are powerful antioxidants, while others have beneficial hormone-like actions or anti-inflammatory effects in the body. They include the following.

Flavonoids These natural antioxidants help to maintain health and protect against disease. As antioxidants, they protect cell membranes from damage, and also help to prevent hardening and furring up of the arteries. Almost every fruit and vegetable contains flavonoids, of which over 20,000 are known to exist. One study found that men who ate the most flavonoids had less than half the number of fatal heart attacks compared with those who ate the least. The chief sources of flavonoids in the study were apples, onions and tea.

Soluble fibre This kind of fibre (see also page 88) keeps the bowels working normally. A number of studies have found that those eating more fruit are less likely to suffer from cancer of the colon. Fibre also has beneficial effects on the absorption of dietary fat.

84

Micronutrients Micronutrients include all the important vitamins, minerals and trace elements you need. Fruit and veg are good sources of the antioxidant vitamins C and E, betacarotene and the mineral selenium. Fruit also contains potassium, which helps to flush excess sodium through the kidneys and may help to reduce high blood pressure.

Phytochemicals These are plant chemicals that seem to help protect against cancer by blocking enzymes needed for the growth of cancer cells.

Phytoestrogens These plant hormones have a weak oestrogen-like effect in the body. This is useful for both men and women as isoflavones interact with oestrogen receptors within the circulation to mimic some of the beneficial effects of oestrogen, helping to dilate coronary arteries, increase heart function, reduce blood levels of harmful LDL cholesterol and reduce blood stickiness to prevent unwanted clotting. These findings may help to explain why the Japanese have one of the lowest rates of coronary heart disease in the world.

Phytoestrogens also have beneficial antioxidant and anti-inflammatory actions which may reduce the risk of atherosclerosis. Based on scientific evidence from over 50 independent studies, the US Food and Drug Administration stated in October 1999 that it will authorise health claims on food labels that 'A diet low in saturated fat and cholesterol, and which includes 25g soya protein per day, can significantly reduce the risk of coronary heart disease'. Soy is also a rich source of protein, calcium and fibre.

What is a serving of fruit or veg?

A serving or portion of fruit and vegetables is best thought of as the amount you are happy to eat in one sitting. Typically, this would amount to:

- a glass of fruit juice
- a large mixed salad
- 1 large beef tomato or 2 medium tomatoes
- a handful of grapes, cherries or berries
- a single apple, orange, kiwi, peach, pear, nectarine or banana
- $\frac{1}{2}$ grapefruit, $\frac{1}{2}$ ogen melon, $\frac{1}{2}$ mango, $\frac{1}{2}$ papaya

- 2 to 4 dates, figs, satsumas, passion fruits, apricots, plums or prunes
- a handful of nuts
- a generous helping of green or root vegetables (excluding potatoes).

As you are now paying attention to the GL (page 72) of fruits and vegetables, you'll have some idea of the ones to go for. But you need to eat fruit and veg that are both low in GL, and high in antioxidants. Chapter 8 delves into these in depth; for now, suffice to say that you have quite a range to choose from – broccoli, carrots, peas, sweet potatoes, watercress, melon, strawberries and kiwi being but a handful. The benefits of eating low-GL fruits and vegetables are so great that some experts now recommend increased intakes of them, as well as antioxidant-rich green and black tea and red wine (see below), over the classic low-cholesterol, low-saturated fat diet.

Tea

Tea is drunk all over the world – Russia, India, the Far and Middle East, Central Asia, the US and, of course, the UK. White, green and black tea are all made from the young leaves and leaf buds of the same shrub, *Camellia sinensis*.

Green tea is made by steaming and drying fresh tea leaves immediately after harvesting, while black tea is made by crushing and fermenting the freshly cut tea leaves so they oxidise before drying. This allows natural enzymes in the tea leaves to produce the characteristic red-brown colour and relative lack of astringency. White tea is similar to green tea, as it's not fermented, but it is made using only new tea buds, picked before they open. These appear white because they're covered in fine, silvery hairs. The buds are gently dried and make a straw-coloured tea that lacks the characteristic 'grassy' flavour of green tea. White tea also contains less caffeine than other varieties – around 15mg per cup, compared to 20mg for green tea and 40mg for black tea.

Whatever the type, tea is an antioxidant powerhouse. Over 30 per cent of the dry weight of green tea leaves, for instance, consists of powerful flavonoid antioxidants such as catechins. Green tea extracts have an antioxidant action at least 100 times more powerful than vitamin C, and 25 times more powerful than vitamin E.

Drinking white, green or black tea has beneficial effects on blood pressure, blood lipids and blood stickiness, and can lower the risk of developing coronary heart disease and stroke. Those drinking at least four cups of tea a day are half as likely to have a heart attack as non-tea drinkers. A high tea intake (such as eight to 10 cups per day) may also reduce the risk of some cancers.

As even white tea does contain some caffeine, drinking this amount of tea may have an effect on blood glucose levels (although the evidence for this is not robust); but the antioxidant benefits outweigh the risks. For those who wish to avoid caffeine, an excellent substitute is Redbush or rooibosch tea, made from the leaves of a South African shrub. It is naturally free from caffeine and contains less than half the tannin found in regular black tea. Research suggests it provides health benefits in the form of antioxidant, anti-inflammatory, anti-spasmodic and anti-allergy activity. It can be drunk with or without milk, sugar or lemon.

Alcohol

It is refreshing to know that wine – that ancient, pleasurable drink – can be good for us, in moderation at least. Many studies have found that a moderate intake of alcohol reduces the risk of coronary heart disease by as much as 40 per cent. Red wine seems particularly beneficial, especially if drunk with meals.

Red wine contains many compounds with natural antioxidant action, which can raise levels of protective HDL cholesterol and inhibit blood clot formation. Moderate drinkers (those consuming two to three units of alcohol per day) have a lower blood pressure, less risk of a stroke, and less chance of developing serious atherosclerosis than non-drinkers, as well as a lower incidence of coronary heart disease. In a study involving 129,000 people, drinking wine was associated with a significantly lower risk of cardiovascular death (30 per cent less for men, 40 per cent for women) when compared with drinking spirits.

But the beneficial effects of alcohol must be weighed up against the bad. It's all in *how* you handle your tipple. If you binge-drink at weekends, you'll have almost twice the risk of sudden cardiovascular death, due to heart rhythm abnormalities, than moderate or non-drinkers. Men who regularly drink six units of alcohol per day (that's six glasses of wine or three pints of normal-strength beer) are more likely to have a heart attack than those who drink within recommended limits. In any case, as you will be aware, having diabetes means you must watch your alcohol consumption carefully.

This doesn't mean abstinence. People with diabetes may drink alcohol in moderation, just like everyone else. In practice, this means a weekly maximum of no more than 2 to 3 units of alcohol per day for women (3 to 4 for men) with, overall, no more than 14 units per week for women (21 for men). Aim to have at least two alcohol-free days every week, if not more. When you do drink, it may be wise to stick to just one or two glasses of wine per day, and to aim to avoid spirits and beer if you have diabetes.

Alcohol does lower blood glucose levels and it is important to know that, if you drink too much, you may be less aware than usual of the symptoms of an impending hypoglycaemic attack. To help maintain blood glucose levels, only drink after you have eaten a meal and have a low-GL snack while drinking. Have a snack before bedtime too, and keep a close eye on your glucose levels via extra monitoring.

A unit of alcohol is smaller than you might think. One unit (10g alcohol) is equivalent to:

= 100ml wine (one small glass) or

= 50ml sherry (one measure) or

= 25ml spirit (one tot) or

= 300ml beer ($^1/_2$ pint).

Fibre: regulating insulin

Fruit and vegetables, as we've seen, give you a lot of crucial high-quality antioxidants. They also contain another substance vital to diabetic health: fibre. Diabetes has been linked with an inadequate fibre intake, so getting enough of it is very important.

There are two main types of dietary fibre: soluble and insoluble.

Soluble fibre comes into its own in the stomach and upper intestines, where it forms a kind of gel that slows down digestion and absorption – especially of carbohydrates – and so helps blunt the rise in blood glucose level after a meal. Taking fibre supplements such as guar gum or pectin with meals, for example, has been shown to have a beneficial effect on blood glucose control in people with diabetes, reducing both insulin requirements and glucose lost in urine.

Insoluble fibre is more important in the large bowel. It bulks up the faeces, absorbs water and hastens stool excretion. In general, soluble fibre is totally broken down in the large bowel, while insoluble fibre is passed out in the motions.

All plant foods contain both soluble and insoluble fibre, though some sources are richer in one type than another. For instance, wheat and rice bran, celery, fruit and vegetable skins, nuts and seeds are all rich in insoluble fibre, while fruits such as pears, starchy and other vegetables, oats, barley, flaxseed, beans, lentils, peas and soy products such as tofu all contain abundant soluble fibre. Good 'crossover' high-fibre foods, which contain both kinds, include oats, flaxseeds and fruit and vegetables.

With such a wide variety of fibre-rich foods, increasing your fibre intake should be easy. For instance, you could eat porridge for breakfast twice a week, snack on a handful of walnuts or sunflower seeds, make a pot of lentil soup for dinner, ensure you eat apples and pears unpeeled. If you haven't been eating much fibre, though, it's important to give yourself about a week and increase the amount you're eating slowly, to help your intestines adapt. Drink plenty of fluids, and add in a probiotic supplement (page 117) to ensure a healthy balance of bacteria to help process fibre in the lower bowel. Even when following a low-carbohydrate diet, it is important that you get a minimum of five servings of fruit and vegetables a day for their fibre content, or to take fibre supplements such as sterculia, bran or ispaghula (psyllium). Fibre supplements are best changed every few weeks, as bowel bacteria tend to adapt to them.

Salt: handle with care

Do you know how much salt you eat? It's not always easy to gauge, because of the amount of 'hidden' salt in processed food, added to enhance its flavour, act as a stabiliser and preservative, and retain moisture. But it is important: eating too much salt is implicated in high blood pressure, heart disease and stroke.

Studies have suggested that not adding salt during cooking, or at the table, can lower your blood pressure by at least 5mmHg. By reducing your salt intake from 9g a day to 6g, you can lower your risk of a stroke by 22 per cent and your risk of death from coronary heart disease by 16 per cent.

But what can we do about hidden salt, which makes up three-quarters of our daily intake? Most of this is found in tinned products such as soups and sauces, packaged bread, ready meals, biscuits, cakes and breakfast cereals. When you consider that the recommended daily intake of salt is less than 6g per day, while a typical microwave meal provides around 5g, a bowl of breakfast cereal contains 1g and a bowl of canned soup gives 2g, you can see it easily mounts up to the daily intake for the average UK adult of around 9g salt.

So cutting back shouldn't be all that difficult – you just need to avoid processed and salty foods, or in the case of bread and tinned foods such as tuna or soup, peruse the label for salt content. (When reading labels, salt content given as 'sodium' needs to be multiplied by 2.5 to give the equivalent amount of table salt: thus, a serving of soup containing 0.4g sodium contains 1g salt.). Also, avoid or severely limit:

• obviously salty foods such as crisps, bacon and salted nuts
• products canned in brine
• cured, smoked or pickled fish/meats
• meat pastes, pâtés
• stock cubes and yeast extracts.

If you're worried about food tasting too bland without added salt, now is the perfect time to start experimenting with herbs, spices and other taste enhancers, such as lime juice (wonderful with fruit salads, in salad dressings and squeezed into chicken broth, for example). It doesn't take long to retrain your taste buds.

Where salt is essential, use mineral-rich rock salt rather than table salt, or a low-sodium, higher-potassium brand of salt sparingly (these can taste bitter). Potassium is valuable as it helps to flush excess sodium from the body via the kidneys, and a diet that is lacking in potassium is linked with a higher risk of high blood pressure and stroke, especially if your diet is also high in sodium. In one study, people taking medication for high blood pressure were able to reduce their drug dose by half (under medical supervision) after increasing the potassium content of their food. Sodium and potassium are covered in detail on page 187.

Children can tolerate less sodium than adults, yet are subjected to an onslaught of it in popular children's snacks such as crisps. It's important to limit their salt intake; the box below provides guidelines.

How much salt for children?

In 2003, the Food Standards Agency announced target maximum intakes for children.

Age	Target salt intake (g per day maximum)
0 to 6 months	less than 1
7–12 months	1
1–3 years	2
4–6 years	3
7–10 years	5
from age 11 onwards	6 (as for adults)

6

Losing weight

By now, we've seen that obesity and overweight are the biggest risk factors for diabetes, particularly if the excess weight builds up around the midriff – the so-called apple shape. So if you are very overweight, have metabolic syndrome or have been diagnosed as having type 2 diabetes, choosing a workable, healthy weight loss diet and exercise regime should be a top priority.

By shedding excess pounds, you can reduce your risk of developing type 2 diabetes by over 50 per cent and, if you already have diabetes, significantly lower your chance of developing diabetic complications. In fact, if you're overweight and have type 2 diabetes, each kilogram of weight lost within a year of being diagnosed can lengthen your life by three to four months. That's a whole extra year of life for each 3kg to 4kg excess weight you can lose. And losing 10 per cent of your body weight – 10kg (22lb), for someone weighing 100kg (15 stone 8lb) – can:

• reduce the chance of diabetes-related death by 30 per cent
• halve fasting blood glucose levels
• allow blood pressure to fall by as much as 10/10mmHg
• reduce fasting triglyceride levels by 30 per cent
• lower total cholesterol by 10 per cent
• lower harmful LDL cholesterol by 15 per cent
• increase beneficial HDL cholesterol by 8 per cent.

But dramatic as these benefits are, it is vital that you seek advice from your doctor before starting any weight-loss diet, especially if you are using medication to control your diabetes. You may need to reduce the dose of some of your medications or even stop taking them if you're cutting back on the amount you eat, and especially if you choose to follow a low-carbohydrate diet. Any diet you follow will need to be tailored to your own very special circumstances.

You will also need to remember to monitor your blood glucose levels frequently, and ensure you eat enough to avoid hypoglycaemia. So be aware that the information in this chapter is general only, and has to be viewed as secondary to the advice of your own doctor.

We'll be looking at the various kinds of weight-loss diets in this chapter. But the food itself is only part of the story. The other part lies in *how* we eat. There are all sorts of ways in which you can make weight loss easier – even pleasurable!

Tips on how to eat less

- Drink a large glass of sparkling mineral water before every meal – this will make you feel full more quickly, so you eat less.
- If possible, try to eat the main meal of the day at lunchtime. Your metabolic rate is higher then than in the evening, so more calories are burned than converted into fat. Try not to eat late at night.
- Always sit down at a table to eat – don't eat while standing up.
- Serve smaller helpings than you think you need.
- Use a smaller plate than usual.
- Eat as slowly as possible, so that metabolic messages that you are full start to come through before you have finished wolfing down your food:
  - Chew each mouthful longer than usual.
  - Pause regularly while eating and put down your knife and fork between bites.
  - Rediscover the art of mealtime conversation.
- Concentrate on enjoying your food. Don't read or watch TV at the same time – you will swallow mechanically without appreciating your food and end up eating more.
- Try not to eat while driving – this can become a habit on long journeys.
- When you feel the urge to eat between meals, do some vigorous

---

exercise and work up a sweat – or try cleaning your teeth with strong, tingling toothpaste.

- If you need a snack to help maintain blood glucose levels, select a healthy option such as a small handful of nuts or seeds, a piece of low-GL fruit, or an oatcake with cottage cheese, for example.
- Keep a food diary and write down everything you eat if the scales refuse to budge.

Types of weight-loss diet

There are four main types of weight-loss diet:
- low-calorie diets, which typically provide 1000 to 1500kcals a day
- very low-calorie diets, which usually provide 400 to 1000kcals a day
- low-fat diets, which typically provide less than 30 per cent of daily energy as fat
- low-carbohydrate diets (which tend to provide 20 to 120g carbo-hydrate daily, depending on your personal carbohydrate toler-ance level).

We'll be looking at each below in terms of how well they actu-ally work. As you will see, I believe – based on all the available evidence so far – that low-carbohydrate diets, and particularly the Atkins-style diet, are the most effective at promoting weight loss especially for people with metabolic syndrome or diabetes type 2. But let's weigh up the evidence.

Low-calorie diets

A low-calorie diet will help you lose weight, as long as you're able to follow it long-term. Many people start out on such diets with the best intentions, but fail to persist because they become bored or hungry. Counting calories can be time-consuming and it is easy to underestimate the amount eaten. Ideally, you should weigh foods at the beginning as this will help you get used to gauging, for example, the size of a piece of cheese containing 120kcals of energy.

On average, people following a low-calorie diet lose around

8 per cent of their body weight over 6 to 12 months. For someone weighing 100kg, that would be 8kg. Studies looking at the long-term outcomes of low-calorie diets, and dieters' ability to keep weight off after following them, suggest they are less effective, however. After 3 to 4 years, the average weight loss is half that seen in shorter-term trials, at around 4 per cent of body weight – equivalent to just 4kg for someone who starts out weighing 100kg.

Very low-calorie diets

With very low-calorie diets or VLCDs, you usually drink a nutritionally complete vitamin and mineral enriched liquid formula in the form of a sweet or savoury shake/soup mix. This can be used to replace one, two or even all of the main meals of the day.

VLCDs prescribed in a clinical setting (with professional support from a trained counsellor, nurse or doctor) and providing as little as 400 to 500kcals per day are more effective for rapid weight loss than a standard low-calorie diet. On average, people will lose 13 to 23kg excess weight on them. After one year, however, there is little difference in the amount of weight lost from following a VLCD or a low-calorie diet.

Sometimes people use a VLCD for a period of up to four weeks, to kickstart a longer-term diet plan. They can, however, be followed for a year or more, as long as you are closely supervised by someone trained in this method of weight loss. In fact, an overview of 29 studies investigating how well people managed to keep excess weight off once they had lost it found that VLCDs helped more people keep off significantly more weight at every year of follow-up – even up to five years.

VLCDs have been used successfully by people with diabetes and can produce a more rapid weight loss than a conventional low-fat diet.

Some expert bodies, such as the American Diabetes Association, suggest that VLCDs are suitable for anyone with a body mass index (page 54) above $25kg/m^2$, which indicates they are over-weight or obese. Others, including the European Association for the Study of Diabetes, suggest they are more suitable for people with a BMI greater than $35kg/m^2$, meaning they are very obese.

VLCDs should only be used as part of an ongoing, structured education and behavioural support programme designed to help you change your long-term eating and lifestyle habits. Close support is essential to help you stick to the very restricted diet and to help you reintroduce normal foods once you have lost your goal weight. It's also vitally important to seek medical advice regarding your medication, if you take any, as you will have much less energy than normal on this diet. You will probably need to have your dose reduced, and you must also monitor your blood glucose levels carefully.

Conventional low-fat diets

For people needing to lose a fair bit of weight, most doctors and traditionally trained dieticians recommend a conventional low-fat, high-fibre diet. The International Task Force for managing coronary risk factors in people with diabetes recommend following a diet that supplies 55 per cent total calories as carbohydrate, and that total fat should be restricted to 30 per cent or less of daily energy, with saturated fat reduced to less than 7 per cent of that total. They encourage moderate consumption of monounsaturated fats such as olive and rapeseed oils, and polyunsaturated fats like fish or flaxseed oils, but say refined and processed carbohydrates such as simple sugars should be severely restricted.

Originally, low-fat diets were based on the idea that because fat supplies twice as many calories per gram as either protein or carbohydrate, cutting back on it will cut back on calorie intake more effectively than cutting back on other food groups. However, there is conflicting evidence about the effectiveness of the low-fat approach to weight loss.

It seems that low-fat diets are no better than low-calorie diets in helping people to lose weight over the long term, and that it's the restriction on overall calories that promotes weight loss rather than the restriction of fat alone. Often, people following a low-fat diet lose no more than 3 to 4kg. This is partly because low-fat diets are unpalatable and difficult to follow, and partly because you eat more carbohydrates when you're on them. This actually impedes weight loss. Carbohydrate triggers the production of insulin in people whose pancreas is still producing it, or requires insulin injections or hypoglycaemic drugs in the rest. Insulin, however, switches off the fat-burning mechanisms in the body and promotes fat storage – so the result is the exact opposite of what you are trying to achieve!

Low fat, low efficacy

A 2002 review of low-fat diets for the obese, produced by the nonprofit healthcare review body the Cochrane Collaboration, looked at all the available randomised clinical trials comparing low-fat diets with other weight loss approaches. This included 4 studies lasting 6 months each, 5 year-long studies, and 3 studies that included 18 months of follow-up.

In the six-month studies the reviewers found no significant difference in weight loss between those following a low-fat diet and control groups following low-calorie diets. Average weight loss was 5.08kg in those following a low-fat diet and 6.5kg in the control groups – showing that those who followed a low-fat diet did worse than those who didn't. In the year-long studies, average weight loss in the low-fat group was just 2.3kg, compared with a loss of 3.4kg in the control group. In the studies with 18-month follow-ups, the average weight loss in those in the control groups was again 2.3kg. But those following a low-fat diet had actually gained 0.1kg, so were marginally heavier than when they had started trying to lose weight a year and a half previously! Not impressive.

Overall, there were no significant differences between the groups in blood fat levels, blood pressure or fasting glucose levels. The conclusion was that a low-fat diet is no better than a low-calorie diet for helping overweight or obese people lose excess weight.[10]

Why do doctors and dieticians continue to recommend a high-carbohydrate, low-fat diet? It's something of a mystery, as this way of eating is known to impair glucose tolerance, increase triglyceride levels and decrease HDL cholesterol concentration if they are not highly enriched with fibre.[11,12,13]

Low-carbohydrate diets

As we've seen, the low-fat approach to weight loss has not worked. Having reviewed all the clinical evidence, I now believe that a low-carbohydrate approach to weight loss is a far more effective way to lose excess weight, and is the preferred approach for most people, including those with metabolic syndrome and type 2 diabetes. This is because it works with your body's own biochemistry and metabolism to help burn excess fat, rather than striving to store it.

Unfortunately, most doctors, dieticians and nutritionists have a knee-jerk reaction against low-carbohydrate diets – usually because they know little about them and have not reviewed the evidence. However, well-controlled, peer-reviewed research has shown that following a diet that limits carbohydrates results in greater weight loss, increased 'good' HDL cholesterol and significantly reduced triglyceride levels in most people who follow them. In fact, for people with diabetes who have raised triglyceride levels and raised LDL cholesterol, there is now a move towards recommending a lower-carbohydrate, high-monounsaturated fat diet in which 60 to 70 per cent of total energy is divided between monounsaturated fat (such as olive and rapeseed oil) and carbohydrate to more closely mimic the Mediterranean diet.

One study, published in the *Journal of the American Medical Association*,[14] found that people with type 2 diabetes who switched between a lower-carbohydrate, high-monounsaturated fat diet and a higher carbohydrate diet experienced a persistent improvement in glycaemic control and lowered high insulin levels on the one with lower carbohydrate levels. The conclusion from a meta-analysis of this approach was that, compared with high-carbohydrate diets, diets high in monounsaturated fat improve blood fat levels as well as blood glucose control.[15]

The controlled carbohydrate diet developed by the late Dr Robert Atkins, now known as the Atkins Nutritional Approach, appears to be an even more effective way for people with metabolic syndrome and type 2 diabetes to lose excess weight. Certainly, of all the low-carb diets currently on offer, it has the most scientific research to back it up.

The Atkins approach

You'll probably have heard of the Atkins diet, which encourages the body to burn fat rather than glucose. In the last decade its popularity has skyrocketed, yet it remains highly controversial among many members of the medical community, partly because they feel (wrongly) that its relatively high-fat content could contribute to heart disease. In fact, this is not borne out by research. We'll examine some of the scientific evidence backing the diet later in this chapter and in Appendix 3.

I advocate the Atkins diet because it works, and its efficacy and safety is supported by extensive research. But if you have type 2 diabetes and choose to embark on it, it's essential that you follow it under the supervision of a doctor or nutritionist who is well versed in the method. If you are on medication to lower your blood glucose levels, this will usually need to be changed before you begin a low-carb diet. You must not do this on your own, but to give you an idea of what your doctor might advise, usually most oral tablets except metformin are stopped, and insulin doses are usually reduced or (if you are on a low daily amount) may even be stopped as you adopt the low-carb approach. You must monitor your blood glucose level carefully and follow instructions from your doctor about how to adjust your dose(s) as your blood glucose level comes down.

When you're ready to start, first off, you will need to buy the book – *Dr Atkins New Diet Revolution* (Vermilion) or *Atkins for Life – The Next Level* (Macmillan). And you'll have to follow the instructions carefully. This means working through the programme from the beginning; remembering to drink at least 2 litres of water a day; taking the recommended supplements; and eating regularly, without skipping meals.

If you are on medication to lower your blood glucose levels, this will usually need to be changed before you begin the diet. You must monitor your blood glucose level carefully and follow instructions from your doctor about how to adjust your dose(s) as your blood glucose level comes down.

What to expect on Atkins Let's say you've just begun the Atkins Nutritional Approach. In the initial 'induction' phase you'll restrict the carbohydrates that affect your blood glucose levels to 20g per day by avoiding refined white bread, potatoes and sugars, but still obtaining fibre and the high-quality carbohydrates found in many vegetables. The induction phase lasts for a minimum of two weeks, during which your body switches from primarily burning glucose for fuel, to mainly burning fat. This produces a metabolic state known as benign dietary ketosis (see box). If you have a lot of weight to lose, or if you seem to lose weight slowly, you may decide to stick to the induction phase for longer – some people stay in it for six months or more.

Ketones and ketosis

Ketones are the basic form in which the body obtains energy from fatty acids, just as glucose is the basic form in which the body obtains energy from carbohydrates. The liver makes three different ketones (acetoacetate, hydroxybutyrate and acetone) from fatty acids and from some amino acids. After an overnight fast, most people produce some ketones as their liver will have used up all its spare carbohydrate (glycogen) stores, and will start burning fat and producing ketones for energy instead.

Once ketones reach tissues in need of energy, such as muscle cells, they are transported into the mitochondria (the cells' energy-producing 'factories') where they are oxidised to produce energy, just like other breakdown products of carbohydrate, protein and fat metabolism. As ketones are water soluble, some are lost from the body in urine and can be detected on urinalysis sticks (such as Ketostix). As ketones are also volatile, they are sometimes detectable on the breath.

When following a low-carbohydrate diet, ketone levels usually remain relatively low at 1 to 3mmol/l, and may even be undetectable in someone with obesity and/or metabolic syndrome or type 2 diabetes. It is important not to confuse this mild, benign dietary ketosis with ketoacidosis – a potentially life-threatening condition that occurs in someone with uncontrolled diabetes (see page 37). Ketoacidosis is associated with very high levels of ketones, which can build up in the blood to a level greater than 20mmol/l in people whose metabolism is very abnormal because of very high blood levels of glucose. As cells cannot access this glucose in someone with untreated diabetes, because of a lack of insulin, they are forced to change their metabolism and produce lots of lactic and other acids, which build up to overwhelm the body's normal buffering mechanisms. This abnormal metabolism and high levels of glucose also lead to dehydration, and can lead to ketoacidosis. It is the excess acid, glucose and dehydration that are harmful, rather than the ketones themselves.

In contrast, benign dietary ketosis is a regulated and controlled production of ketones in the body brought about by following a low-carbohydrate diet. It's associated with relatively normal levels of glucose, acids and hydration levels.

If you have type 2 diabetes or metabolic syndrome and are following a low-carb diet, low levels of ketones in your urine are not harmful *as long as your glucose levels are well-controlled, and you are well hydrated from drinking plenty of water.* In fact, by following a low-carbohydrate diet, your blood glucose control should improve significantly. If you are uncertain about this point, however, it is important to seek clarification from a medical doctor who is well versed in the science behind low-carbohydrate diets.

Remember: if you have diabetes or metabolic syndrome, your metabolism is abnormal, and it is important to follow a low-carbohydrate diet *only* with supervision from a doctor who's familiar with the programme, and who can adjust your medication and tell you how to change your dose as your condition comes under better control.

If you are diabetic and detect very high levels of ketones in your urine, or if your glucose control seems to be poor, seek immediate medical advice.

The next phase of the Atkins programme, known as ongoing weight loss, allows you to slowly increase the amount of carbohydrates you eat by 5g per day for each week. The first week you will have 25g carbohydrate per day, the second week you'll have 30g per day, and so on until you find your weight loss slows. You then drop back by 5g of carbohydrate per day to the previous level, as this represents the amount of carbohydrate you can eat per day while still continuing to lose weight slowly.

When adding carbohydrates back in to your diet, you first eat more salad and other vegetables, then more cheese, nuts, seeds and berries. As you keep adding in more carbohydrates, you can start to eat legumes and fruits other than berries, working up the Atkins carbohydrate ladder to reintroduce a few starchy vegetables and even some wholegrains until you find the level at which you stop losing weight slowly. It is a myth that you don't get any fruit and vegetables while following a low-carbohydrate diet. You still need to have five servings a day, in the form of salad leaves, peppers, tomatoes, avocado, broccoli, spinach, asparagus, green beans, mushrooms, celery and so on.

During this phase you can also drink a little dry wine, spirits and other low-carb alcoholic beverages, if you wish. A range of low-carb snacks and shakes are now also available, sweetened with substances having a minimal effect on blood sugar levels, such as glycerine, maltitol and sucralose. The only carbs you count are those that significantly affect your blood glucose levels, and these are referred to on Atkins products and in their carbohydrate gram counters as 'net carbs'.

Once you come within about 5kg or 10lb of your target weight, you enter the third phase of the Atkins programme, known as the pre-maintenance phase. At this point you add in more grams of daily carbohydrate intake at a rate of 5 to 10g per week, as long as you still continue to lose weight slowly at an almost imperceptible rate (such as 1lb per month). Once you have reached your goal weight, and maintained it for one month, you will know the level of carbohydrates you can eat per day without gaining or losing weight. This is referred to as your Atkins carbohydrate equilibrium or ACE.

You then enter the fourth phase, lifetime maintenance, in which you continue to eat a controlled carbohydrate diet according to your own personal ACE. The amount of carbohydrate you can eat daily varies from person to person but is usually within 40 and 120g per day.

Other low-carbohydrate diets are available, such as The Zone, The New High Protein Diet and the South Beach Diet, but these have not been subject to as much research as the Atkins approach and are really just variations on the general theme.

For more information on the Atkins Nutritional Approach, visit www.atkins.com/uk. A new book, *The Atkins Diabetes Revolution* (Thorsons), is also available. This goes into the science between low-carb diets and diabetes in much more detail.

In the US, many doctors now advocate a low-carbohydrate approach to help people with metabolic syndrome and type 2 diabetes lose weight, lower their insulin levels, reduce their insulin resistance, lower their blood pressure, reduce their triglyceride levels, lower their LDL cholesterol and raise their HDL cholesterol – in effect, reversing all the findings associated with metabolic syndrome and lowering their risk of heart disease and stroke. Doctors in the UK have been slower in understanding that it is a high-carbohydrate diet that fuels metabolic syndrome and type 2 diabetes. At the same time, many doctors still fear that people eating a diet that provides more fat than usual will increase the risk of coronary heart disease, although this is not the case.

The evidence for the Atkins way of eating Many studies have now shown the effectiveness of the Atkins low-carbohydrate approach in triggering weight loss and helping to combat metabolic syndrome and type 2 diabetes.

For example, when over 75,000 women aged between 38 and 63, with no previous history of diabetes, angina, heart attack or stroke, were followed for 10 years from 1984, the amount of carbohydrate they ate was found to be directly associated with their risk of developing coronary heart disease after taking age, smoking status, total energy intake, and other known coronary heart disease risk factors into account.[16] Those with the highest intake of carbohydrate had twice the risk of a heart attack compared to those with the lowest intake.

A number of studies have now also compared low-carb with low-fat/low-calorie diets in randomised controlled trials, and the most important of these – some involving people with diabetes and metabolic syndrome – are reviewed in Appendix 3 (page 249). You can find abstracts of these studies at www.atkins.com/uk.

These studies all provide important information for doctors caring for people who are obese, especially if they also have metabolic syndrome or type 2. If your doctor dismisses your request to supervise you while following a low-carb diet, please suggest that they obtain these papers and read them as part of their continuing medical education.

If they are worried about all the myths they have heard concerning the so-called 'dangers' of following a low-carbohydrate diet, I suggest they read Anssi Manninen's recent review in the *Sports Nutrition Review Journal*, 'High-protein weight loss diets and purported adverse effects: Where is the evidence?' (*Sports Nutr Rev J* 1(1)45–51, 2004; available online at www.sportsnutrtion society.org/site/admin/pdf/Manninen%20SNRJ%201-1-45-51-2004.pdf). Manninen, a member of the medical faculty at the University of Oulu in Finland, finds that there is no basis to the claim that low-carb, high-protein diets cause potential abnormalities in the bones, liver, heart or kidneys, as long as these are healthy in the first place.

Boost that metabolism: the importance of exercise

Eating the right foods is a vital part of the weight-loss equation. The other is exercise. Exercise is the most effective known way to increase your metabolic rate (as much as tenfold). It boosts fat loss by increasing the movement of fatty acids out of fat cells and increasing their availability as a fuel for muscle cells, helping you to lose weight. Research has also shown, for example, that when you walk briskly and steadily for some time, your blood fat levels will rise much less than usual after eating, as dietary fats are rapidly burned for fuel rather than added to fat stores. This effect was noticed even when participants exercised up to 15 hours before a meal, or 90 minutes after it.

Even if you don't change your eating habits, increasing your level of physical activity will help you lose weight. If you start to exercise for 45 minutes to an hour a day, you can shed a modest 2 to 3kg in a month. Walking briskly, at about 4.5 miles per hour, for 30 minutes can also burn 200 extra calories – enough to lose a pound every two weeks if you did this every day. Diet plus exercise is usually more effective than either approach alone although, surprisingly, the evidence for this is conflicting. It does seem, however, that exercise helps people to lose fat around their waistline which, as we've seen, is the 'danger zone' for fat storage. People who exercise regularly are also more likely to keep off the weight they have lost than those who exercise less.

Aim to exercise briskly (walking, swimming, cycling, jogging, gym work) for at least half an hour every day. If you're unfit, start off slowly and increase the amount of effort you put into it as you become more fit.

For further information – including reviews of the research available – on how exercise can reduce your risk of developing type 2 diabetes, see Appendix 1. Note that if you're using medication to reduce blood glucose levels, you will need to discuss your monitoring of blood glucose levels with your doctor, as you may have to do it more frequently, as well as adjust your medication when following an exercise and/or diet regime. Monitor your blood glucose before and after exercise and make sure you have immediate access to a rapidly absorbed form of carbohydrate (such as 55ml of a high-energy glucose drink or 100ml of cola) in case you start to develop hypoglycaemia. You can usually avoid a hypo by planning exercise sessions and reducing your dose of medication beforehand. After intensive exercise, you may also need to reduce your drug dose and have extra food.

It's usually recommended that you postpone exercise if your blood glucose concentration is above 15mmol/l, and that you should have additional carbohydrate if your blood glucose levels are less than 7mmol/l. If you're in any doubt at all about how much exercise to take, or how it will affect your diabetes, seek medical advice from your doctor.

7

Nutritional supplements: The basics

Vitamins, minerals, trace elements and other micronutrients, such as flavonoids, are not 'little extras' in your diet. Instead, they're the 'X factor' – the substances that keep us in top shape inside and out, glowing with vitality.

Most of the metabolic pathways in your body need vitamins or minerals to work properly, and if an essential micronutrient is lacking, vital regeneration and repair processes will slow down. Vitamin B3, or niacin, for instance, is necessary for brain function and the production of energy, and it also helps balance cholesterol and blood glucose levels – obviously of prime importance if you have diabetes or metabolic syndrome.

In fact, you need a wide range of vitamins, minerals and other micronutrients to keep your blood glucose levels in order. A number of nutritional supplements are key for people with diabetes, countering the harmful process of oxidation in the body, improving the flow and consistency of your blood, reducing the risk of heart attack and stroke, and lessening the effects of complications such as retinopathy or peripheral neuropathy. Yet many of these are commonly in short supply in the typical Western diet. So it's important to choose your food with an eye not just to qualities such as GL, but also to vitamin and mineral content.

However, as I discussed at the start of this book, food storage and processing does leach vitamins from fruit and vegetables. Add to that your need, as a diabetic, for more of certain nutrients, and you can be left wondering about your nutritive status. Are you really getting enough of the nutrients you need? To ensure you do, you need first to concentrate on your diet, and then, supplement as appropriate. In this chapter I concentrate on supplements, but in the chapters that follow I discuss both the foods richest in various micronutrients, as well as the best supplements containing them.

Recommended amounts

If you're new to supplements, the variety on offer in any chemists' or healthfood store may seem completely bewildering. And it's not just the sheer number of combinations and permutations that can seem overwhelming: the amounts of various micronutrients in multivitamin and mineral supplements can also vary significantly. So how much is enough – or too much?

Nutritionists have come up with guidelines that are meant to help us through this maze. Recently, those in the UK have tended to turn away from the old RNI (reference nutrient intake) and adopted equivalents suggested by the European Commission: the recommended daily amount, or RDA. The RDA is an estimated intake believed to supply the needs of up to 97 per cent of the population. (Note that in this book, 'RDA' always refers to the EU RDA unless otherwise indicated.)

Everyone has unique nutritional needs depending on their age, weight, level of activity and the metabolic pathways and enzyme systems they have inherited. Some people will need more of certain nutrients, and some people will need less. In general, having diabetes increases your need for antioxidants (vitamins A, C and E, and selenium) as well as the minerals chromium, zinc and magnesium. The EU RDAs that have been set for labelling purposes can be seen in the table below.

EU RDAs for Vitamins and Minerals

Vitamins	EU RDA
Vitamin A (retinol)	800mcg
Vitamin B1 (thiamin)	1.1mg
Vitamin B2 (riboflavin)	1.4mg
Vitamin B3 (niacin)	16mg

continued overleaf

Vitamin B5 (pantothenic acid)	6mg
Vitamin B6 (pyridoxine)	1.4mg
Vitamin B12 (cyanocobalamin)	2.5mcg
Biotin	50mcg
Folic acid	200mcg*
Vitamin C	80mg
Vitamin D	5mcg
Vitamin E	12mg

* Women planning a baby should take 400mcg.

Minerals	EU RDA
Calcium	800mg
Iodine	150mcg
Iron	14mg
Magnesium	375mg
Phosphorus	700mg
Zinc	10mg

Units of measurement for micronutrients

The vitamins and minerals we need are called micronutrients because – unlike protein, carbohydrates and other 'macronutrients' – we only need them in tiny amounts. The quantities you need are measured in milligrams (mg) or micrograms (mcg).

1 milligram = one thousandth of a gram (1/1000 or 10^{-3} grams)
1 microgram = one millionth of a gram (1/1,000,000 or 10^{-6} grams)
1 milligram therefore = 1000 micrograms.

Vitamin and mineral deficiency

As we've seen, a number of factors militate against our getting enough of the vitamins and minerals we need – food storage and higher requirements for certain micronutrients being two. But many of us are also failing to get enough simply because of poor eating habits. Three-quarters of women and almost 9 out of 10 men eat less than the recommended 5 servings of fruit and vegetables per day. More, over two-thirds of people do not eat oily fish on a regular basis, even though only one or two portions per week will supply all the essential fatty acids they need.

The UK's 2003 National Diet and Nutrition Survey found that the vitamin and mineral intake of significant numbers of men and women lie below the UK RNIs (reference nutrient intakes, which are slightly different from the EC RDAs). So these people are likely to be deficient in these nutrients.

Percentage of Men and Women with Vitamin and Mineral Intake from Food Sources below the UK RNI[17]

Nutrient	Men		Women	
	19–24 yrs (%)	50–64 yrs (%)	19–24 yrs (%)	50–64 yrs (%)
Vitamin A	74	42	81	46
B1	26	10	18	10
B2	40	18	45	8
B3	2	1	4	1
B6	12	7	21	13
B12	4	0	5	1
Folic acid	14	10	40	25
C	39	16	25	12
Iron	25	14	96	38
Calcium	34	14	56	36
Magnesium	76	44	85	66
Zinc	57	41	58	33
Iodine	41	12	63	31
Copper	62	34	78	70

When looking at the *lower* reference nutrient intake (LRNI), which is the amount necessary to prevent a deficiency disease, the results are even more worrying. By this measure, a quarter of all women between the ages of 19 to 64 have seriously low intakes of iron, putting them at risk of iron-deficiency anaemia. Higher numbers of women than expected also have very low intakes of calcium and magnesium.

It is estimated that 60 per cent of the population do not even manage to get 60mg vitamin C per day on a regular basis. And over 90 per cent of the population fail to obtain the recommended 10mg vitamin E. We don't yet have a recommended daily amount for carotenoids, but a minimum intake of 6mg per day (equivalent to 100ml carrot juice) appears to protect against cancer and age-related macular degeneration, an eye condition. Most of us get less than 2mg carotenoids daily from our food.

People trying to lose weight – as many people with metabolic syndrome and diabetes type 2 need to do – are at special risk of deficiencies. The reason is that they are eating less, and unless they're very careful, they will end up consuming fewer vitamins and minerals than non-slimmers. Unfortunately, a number of food surveys have confirmed that this is very much the case.

Generally, however, people seem to be waking up to this problem. More and more of us choose to take a multinutrient supplement as a nutritional safety net, and science is backing up the trend. A review of over 150 clinical trials published in the *Journal of the American Medical Association* in 2002 showed that low intakes of many vitamins is a risk factor for heart disease, stroke, some cancers, birth defects, osteoporosis, bone fractures and other major chronic health problems.[18] In an accompanying paper, the authors say, 'Pending strong evidence of effectiveness from randomised trials, it appears prudent for all adults to take vitamin supplements.'

In the Nurses' Health Study,[19] for example, which began in 1980, more than 80,000 healthy women completed a detailed food questionnaire from which their intake of nutrients could be assessed. Over 14 years of follow-up, the number of heart attacks were recorded as well as factors such as smoking, high blood pressure, and intakes of alcohol, fat and fibre. The researchers found that the risk of coronary heart disease was reduced by around 25 per cent for women who regularly used multivitamin supplements.

Multivitamins and diabetes: major benefits

In the following chapters I'll be going through how specific nutrients can help specific problems or needs arising from diabetes or metabolic syndrome. But even just taking a daily multivitamin and mineral carries significant health benefits.

If you have type 2 diabetes, you may reduce your risk of developing an infection. In one study, 130 people aged from 45 to 64 took a multivitamin and mineral supplement or placebo for one year. Some of them had type 2 diabetes. Some 73 per cent of the people taking a placebo reported an infectious illness over that year, compared with just 43 per cent of those taking the multivitamin and mineral. Infection-related absenteeism was also higher in the placebo group (57 per cent) than in the treated group (21 per cent). What's really remarkable is that these differences were mostly accounted for by participants with type 2 diabetes: out of this group, just 17 per cent who took the multivitamin reported an infection, compared to 93 per cent on the placebo.[20]

Research involving 96 older people has also shown that those taking multivitamins for one year had better immune function, mounted a better response to influenza vaccination, and had half as many days spent ill with infections compared with those not taking multivitamin supplements.

And there's more. A study of 1380 people attending an ophthalmology outpatient clinic found that regular use of multivitamin and antioxidant supplements decreased the risk of developing cataracts by 37 per cent.[21] Cataracts are a significant risk in diabetes, even in children.

Staying safe with vitamins and minerals

There can be too much of a good thing: certain vitamins and minerals are harmful in excess, and it's vital not to exceed the manufacturer's recommended daily dose of any supplement. Safe upper limits for many vitamins and minerals are not yet cast in stone, but the following table provides a good guideline.

Safe Upper Levels for Vitamins and Minerals

Vitamins	Safe upper level for long-term consumption (daily intake)
Vitamin A (retinol)	1500mcg
Vitamin B1 (thiamin)	100mg
Vitamin B2 (riboflavin)	40mg
Vitamin B3 (as nicotinamide)	500mg
Vitamin B5 (pantothenic acid)	200mg
Vitamin B6 (pyridoxine)	10mg
Vitamin B12 (cyanocobalamin)	2000mcg
Biotin	900mcg
Folic acid	1000mcg
Vitamin C	1000mg
Vitamin D	25mcg
Vitamin E	500mg (800IU)
Minerals	
Calcium	1500mg
Iodine	500mcg
Iron	17mg
Magnesium	400mg
Manganese	40mg
Phosphorus	250mg
Zinc	25mg

What to look for in supplements

You can buy supplements in many different forms – tablets, capsules, powders, pastilles, oils, syrups, teas, infusions, effervescent formulations, tinctures and even gels. Generally speaking, the fewer additives, the better. Some will contain sugar as a sweetener, so it is worth checking labels when you are diabetic, and if you are following a low-carbohydrate diet.

But not all additives are harmful. Minerals in tablets are bound (chelated) to other substances, either inorganic salts such as sulphates, carbonates and phosphates, or organic substances such as citrates, fumarates, amino acids and ascorbates. This allows them to pass through the stomach without causing irritation, and helps prevent them from binding with other substances in the digestive tract which would slow or prevent their absorption. In general, better quality supplements contain minerals bound to organic substances as these are more easily digested and absorbed.

Some tablets are made using a time-release process so the active ingredients are delivered at a steady rate over a longer period of time, usually around six hours, rather than all in one go soon after swallowing. This is particularly beneficial for water-soluble vitamins, which the body cannot store.

Checking labels to assess quality

When you read the labels on the jars, they all seem to offer different benefits at different prices – which can simply make the task of choosing the best seem impossible. Labels can, however, help you make your selection. The supplement ingredients – including inactive ingredients such as sugar, colourings and so forth – must be listed in descending order by weight. There will also be a separate nutritional information panel, listing the active ingredients together with their amount and percentage of the recommended daily amount (RDA) where appropriate.

Here are the points you'll need to look for.

- Compare the range of nutrients provided in the supplement – is it a complete 'A to Z' formulation, or does it just provide a few micronutrients, such as B group vitamins? Once you've determined your needs while reading the following chapters, do you find the range of ingredients provided suit them?
- Then compare the amount of each nutrient provided – in the case of vitamins and minerals, this will be compared with the recommended daily amount (RDA). Are they high enough?
- Are minerals chelated with inorganic salts (sulphates, carbonates, phosphates) or organic substances (citrates, amino acids, ascorbates)? The latter tend to be more expensive and better quality.

- Is vitamin E supplied in its natural form, d-alpha tocopheryl, rather than the less active synthetic form, dl-alpha tocopheryl?
- If the supplement contains herbs, are they included as raw powdered herb or as a concentrated extract? Solid extracts are described according to their concentration so that, for example, a 10:1 extract means that 10 parts crude herb was used to make one part of the extract.
- Is the preparation standardised to provide a known and consistent quantity of active ingredients? Non-standardised products could contain very little of the key active components.
- Does the product suit your particular dietary requirements? For example, is it suitable for vegetarians? If you're allergic to a particular substance, such as gluten, yeast, lactose or dairy products, is it free of them?
- Is the product free from artificial sweeteners? Many people prefer to avoid aspartame, for example, especially in children's chewable multivitamin and mineral formulations, although it can be difficult to find any without it!
- How does the price relate to the contents of the product?
- Is it still within its use-by date?
- Check the manufacturer. Is it produced by a well-known, reputable one, whose products are consistently good, and consistently use standardised extracts? (Good-quality products are stocked by the Nutri Centre (tel 0207 323 2382, or www.nutricentre.com) and Healthspan (tel 0800 73 123 77, or www.healthspan.co.uk).

Confusingly, the law states that labels on food supplements are not allowed to carry any claims regarding their effect on health, although there may be agreed statements such as: 'May help to maintain a healthy heart' or 'May help to replenish the vitamin C lost during colds'. Here is where the rest of this book comes into its own. It gives you the information you'll need about the effect of each micronutrient on your health, so you can make sensible and informed choices about supplements.

How to take supplements

If taken on an empty stomach, some vitamin and mineral supplements can make you feel sick or cause indigestion. So they are usually best taken immediately after food and washed down with water.

Don't wash them down with coffee or tea, as these may interfere with absorption. Coffee, for example, can reduce iron absorption from the gut by up to 80 per cent if drunk within an hour of a meal. It also reduces uptake of zinc and is associated with the increased excretion of magnesium, calcium and other minerals. Against this, however, is the fact that caffeine is a potent stimulator of gastric acid secretion, which will assist absorption of some micronutrients such as zinc, whose uptake requires increased acidity. It is also a rich source of vitamin B3, or niacin, although paradoxically, drinking excess coffee depletes vitamin B levels generally.

If you take a one-a-day vitamin and mineral supplement that is not time-released, it is usually better to take it after your evening meal rather than with breakfast. This is because repair processes and mineral flux in your body are greatest at night, when growth hormone is secreted. You're also probably less likely to drink coffee in the evening, so you will avoid any problems with mineral absorption.

If you need to take two or more capsules of the same preparation a day, spread these out if you can to maximise absorption and ensure fewer fluctuations in blood levels, assuming this is convenient. A day's dose is better taken whenever and wherever you remember it, however, rather than staying in the packet.

Note that if you are pregnant or planning to be, or if you are breastfeeding, do not take any supplements unless they are specifically designed for use during pregnancy. Always check with a doctor or pharmacist if you are unsure. Some products, such as those containing vitamin A – cod liver oil, for instance – and most herbs, including aloe vera and agnus castus, should not be taken during pregnancy.

Store supplements in a cool, dry place away from direct heat and light.

They should always be kept out of the sight and reach of children.

When you're ready to take them

If you wish to take a supplement, follow the general rules below.
• Let your doctor know.
• Check for any potential drug-supplement interactions beforehand.
• Do not stop taking any of your prescribed medications unless told to by your usual doctor.
• Only add one or two remedies at a time, at the lowest suggested dose – you can always increase the dose slowly within the recommended dose range, if the supplement does not affect your glucose control.
• Monitor your blood glucose levels closely and try to maintain tight control.
• Always allow at least one week between treatment changes to allow the body to adjust. In some cases, it can take at least three months to assess the effectiveness of a supplement.

Mixing medications with supplements

If you're about to start taking one or two drugs for, say, obesity or glucose control, and are thinking about buying some of the supplements I recommend later in this book, you may be wondering whether all these substances are actually compatible in your body.

It's an important issue. An estimated 41 per cent of adults in the UK take some form of supplement, whether vitamins, minerals, fish oils or herbal remedies, and a third take them on a daily basis. Meanwhile, the number of prescriptions for orthodox medications is also increasing: one in three people who take a food supplement or herbal remedy also take at least one prescribed drug.

Happily, the risk of serious interactions between vitamins, minerals and prescribed drugs is generally low. Most people can safely take a multivitamin and mineral supplement supplying one or two multiples of the RDA. In fact, many drugs (such as oral contraceptives) appear to deplete your body's stores of vitamins and minerals, making supplements even more important. Specialist supplements that supply many times the RDA of a particular nutrient need to be checked out on an individual basis, however, and are best used only under the supervision of a nutritional therapist.

First let's look at the positively beneficial interactions between drugs and supplements. Generally in these interactions, the supplements either offset the potential side effects of certain drugs, or improve their efficacy. Note, however, that you should always check with your doctor or a pharmacist if you want to take a supplement and are already taking a prescribed or over-the-counter drug.

Beneficial interactions

ACE inhibitors and zinc The long-term use of the ACE inhibitor, captopril, to treat high blood pressure or heart failure appears to deplete zinc levels and can lead to a zinc deficiency. This deficiency is a relatively serious one, and can result in hair loss, skin disorders, problems with the immune system and other conditions. It is therefore a good idea for people taking captopril long term to also take a multivitamin and mineral supplement that includes zinc.

Antibiotics and probiotics Probiotics are composed of 'good' bacteria that produce lactic acid, such as Lactobacilli or Bifidobacteria. Found naturally in the large bowel, they encourage healthy digestion. Probiotics come into their own when you need to take antibiotics. As is now well known, antibiotics kill off good bacteria along with all the harmful ones, causing unpleasant digestive upsets such as diarrhoea and can lead to symptoms resembling those of irritable bowel syndrome. So taking probiotics puts back the friendly bacteria, which can then get to work calming your digestion.

Antibiotics and vitamin K People taking antibiotics over the long term, or on a frequent basis, may benefit from also taking a multivitamin and mineral supplying vitamin K. Antibiotics interfere with the blood-clotting action of vitamin K in the body, and also kill probiotic bacteria in the large intestine that produce vitamin K (see above), so supplementing this micronutrient may balance out your levels.

Antibiotics and bromelain Bromelain is a kind of enzyme found in the pineapple plant which has a beneficial effect on digestion. Some evidence suggests that it improves the action of antibiotics (penicillin and erythromycin) in treating a variety of infections. In one trial, 22 out of 23 people who had not previously responded to antibiotics did so once they started taking bromelain as well.

Antacids, vitamins and minerals The long-term use of antacids can interfere with the absorption of nutrients, including folic acid, and possibly copper and phosphate. A multivitamin and mineral supplement is therefore a good idea if you take antacids.

Aspirin, vitamin C and zinc The long-term use of aspirin has been associated with an increased loss of both vitamin C and zinc in urine, and can lead to vitamin C and zinc depletion. Those on long-term aspirin therapy might benefit from taking a daily supplement providing vitamin C and zinc. Non-acidic forms of vitamin C (such as ester C or other buffered ascorbates) will reduce the risk of acid indigestion.

Beta-blockers and co-enzyme Q10 Beta-blockers (used to treat high blood pressure and angina) inhibit enzymes that use co-enzyme Q10 as a co-factor. Studies suggest that some beta-blocker-induced side effects (from propranolol or timolol) can be reduced by taking CoQ10 supplements.

Corticosteroids, calcium and vitamin D Long-term corticosteroid therapy is well known as a trigger for osteoporosis. Good intakes of calcium and vitamin D are vital to help maintain bone density and protect against this debilitating condition.

Oral contraceptives, vitamins and minerals Oral contraceptives appear to deplete body stores of some vitamins and minerals, especially folic acid, magnesium, B1, B2, B3, B6, B12, C and manganese, but may lead to increased levels of iron, and vitamin A. Although the clinical importance of these interactions is unclear, taking an appropriate multivitamin and mineral, or a folic acid and B group supplement, may be sensible.

Paracetamol and milk thistle People taking paracetamol over the long term (such as for arthritis pain) may benefit from taking milk thistle extracts as well, to help maintain levels of protective glutathione in their liver.

SSRIs and Ginkgo Ginkgo has been shown to help overcome sexual dysfunction which can occur in some people treated with SSRI antidepressants.

Statins and co-enzyme Q10 People taking statins to lower raised lipid levels will experience a significant decline in blood levels of co-enzyme Q10, as these drugs block the action of an enzyme involved in the synthesis of co-enzyme Q10 in the body. Supplements supplying CoQ10 are therefore a good idea, and might also help to reduce some of the muscle side effects that can occur as a result of statin therapy.

Topical fungal treatments and Echinacea One study found that in women with vaginal candida, combining Echinacea, taken orally, with topical econazole nitrate cream reduced the rate of recurrence compared with those using the anti-fungal cream alone. As fungal skin infections are common in people with diabetes, this is worth noting.

Tricyclic antidepressants and co-enzyme Q10 Tricyclic anti-depressants interfere with the action of enzymes that use CoQ10 as a co-factor, and it has been suggested that lack of CoQ10 may contribute to the cardiac side effects of this group of drugs.

Potentially harmful drug-micronutrient interactions

Although the risk of a serious interaction between prescribed drugs and supplements is low, and many potential risks are theoretical, the number of interactions identified is on the rise.

It should be said that this is an evolving area: information is limited, and often based on just one case. But where certain drugs are concerned, it is advisable to err on the side of caution. If you are taking warfarin to thin your blood, for example, you need to be particularly careful.

Lab tests and vitamin C Vitamin C can interfere with some laboratory tests used to assess glucose levels in urine, so if taking supplements containing vitamin C, let your doctor know.

Paracetamol and vitamin C High doses of up to 3g of vitamin C have been shown to prolong the time that paracetamol stays in the body. This may be beneficial when paracetamol is taken for occasional pain relief as long as you do not take the two together regularly, when levels of paracetamol may build up – which might have toxic effects on the liver.

Warfarin and...
- *co-enzyme Q10* This is structurally similar to vitamin K and may interact with warfarin activity.
- *vitamin E* High-dose vitamin E thins the blood by inhibiting platelet clumping and vitamin K-dependent clotting factors, so there is a theoretical potential for interaction with warfarin. A clinical trial found no difference in warfarin activity between those taking either vitamin E (up to 1200mg daily) or placebo, however.
- *essential fatty acids* Essential fatty acid supplements such as omega-3 fish oils, cod liver oil, flaxseed oil and evening primrose oils can usually be safely combined with prescription drugs at recommended doses, but they do have anti-clotting properties. So if you're taking warfarin or aspirin, be aware that omega-3s may increase the potential for bleeding, and get advice before taking them.
- *iron, magnesium, zinc* These minerals may bind with warfarin, so they should be taken at least two hours before or after taking warfarin tablets.
- *vitamin K* If you are on warfarin, do not take supplements containing vitamin K unless directed to do so by a doctor, as vitamin K acts as an antidote to warfarin.

When to avoid or limit herbal remedies

Interactions between prescribed drugs and herbal remedies can occur when both act on the same receptor sites (a specific spot on or in a cell that the drug binds to) in the body, or interact with the same metabolic enzymes. The drugs most likely to interact with herbs are those with a narrow range between effective and toxic doses, such as anticoagulants, sedatives and some drugs prescribed to treat heart problems, depression, diabetes, high blood pressure and epilepsy – so if you're taking such drugs, this is an area you need to explore.

It's vital to check with a doctor or pharmacist first to see if there are any known interactions between herbs you want to take and your prescribed drugs – new ones are identified on a regular basis.

St John's wort St John's wort has proven effective in alleviating mild depression. It interacts with a number of drugs, including warfarin, cyclosporin, oral contraceptives, anticonvulsants, digoxin, theophylline, HIV protease inhibitors used to treat AIDS, and antidepressants. With many of these drugs, the herb's primary effect is to reduce blood levels of the drug, which may make it less effective.

With antidepressants, particularly the SSRI (selective serotonin reuptake inhibitor) type, however, St John's wort can boost the effect of the 'happy' brain chemical serotonin. This can lead to serotonin syndrome, a buildup of serotonin in the brain which is potentially harmful.

If you're taking any of the drugs listed above, it would be wise to avoid St John's wort, or take it only on the advice of your doctor. The herb is also contraindicated if you're taking a triptan medication for migraine.

Herbs that interact with warfarin and aspirin A number of herbal remedies are known to interact with warfarin. There is also a potential for interaction between herbs that affect the way blood platelets stick together and warfarin – and possibly aspirin, if taken over the long term – although these reactions are not proven in many cases. These herbs include:
- danshen (a member of the Salvia family), used to help menstrual irregularity and to relieve bruising
- dong quai (*Angelica sinensis*), used to treat menstrual cramps, irregular periods and menopausal symptoms
- garlic
- ginseng
- bilberry
- chamomile
- black cohosh
- ginger
- Pycnogenol® (pine bark extract)
- red clover
- devil's claw
- Ginkgo.

In a handful of cases, people taking Ginkgo biloba extracts – used to increase blood flow in the brain – in combination with warfarin or aspirin have experienced bleeding within the skull (subarachnoid haemorrhage or subdural haematoma). Although ginkgolides found in Ginkgo biloba do stop platelets in the blood – disc-shaped bodies that aid clotting – from sticking together to a degree, these substances are present only in small concentrations, and their effect on platelet aggregation appears to be negligible when Ginkgo is taken at the recommended dose. However, it may be wiser to err on the side of caution and avoid using Ginkgo biloba together with aspirin or warfarin until any possible interactions have been fully investigated.

If you are taking aspirin and want to take a herbal remedy, seek advice from a pharmacist. If there is no definite contraindication to taking them together, you will usually be advised to monitor yourself for any bruising or increased bleeding and to stop taking the herb and seek advice from your doctor if these occur.

Other notable potential herb-drug interactions include:

- diuretics with dandelion, Ginkgo, horsetail, liquorice and uva-ursi
- thyroxine with lemon balm.

8

Antioxidants

Antioxidants are a bit like miniature superheroes in the body. While our body proteins, fats, cell membranes and genetic material are bombarded constantly by free radicals – oxidised molecules in car exhaust, industrial air pollution and other sources – antioxidants are perfectly designed to zap these 'villains' into submission. And in doing so, they protect us from a range of serious health problems common in diabetes: hardening and furring up of the arteries, coronary heart disease, deteriorating vision and impaired immunity. So if you have metabolic syndrome or diabetes, antioxidants are some of your best friends.

There are over a hundred known antioxidants, some recently discovered. As we saw in Chapter 5, many are nutrients found in fruits and vegetables. Tea and red wine contain others, while a number – such as Pycnogenol®, from a species of pine, can only be taken in supplements. The most important dietary antioxidants are:
- polyphenols (flavonoids, anthocyanidins, proanthocyanidins, catechins)
- vitamin A, betacarotene and other carotenoids
- vitamin C
- vitamin E
- selenium.

Lesser antioxidants that are also important include:
- riboflavin
- copper

- manganese
- zinc.

Although diet should always come first, having diabetes means you have a higher need for some antioxidants, making it difficult to get the optimal quantities you require. So while the advice in Chapter 5 is important as a basis for your diet, supplementing antioxidants is a good move – and this chapter contains everything you'll need to know about the best on offer.

The most important antioxidants for people with diabetes are:
- Alpha-lipoic acid, which helps to improve glucose control and insulin sensitivity. It is also helpful for improving symptoms of diabetic nerve damage (polyneuropathy) and may improve kidney function.
- Lutein, a carotenoid related to vitamin A, which helps to protect against age-related macular degeneration.
- Vitamin C, which is involved in the regulation of blood glucose levels, and is also needed to help maintain healthy blood vessels and to reduce formation of a harmful substance (sorbitol) linked with diabetic cell damage.
- Co-enzyme Q10, which improves glucose control in type 2 diabetes, and has beneficial effects on blood vessels which can reduce raised blood pressure. It also helps to reduce the risk of side effects from statins – a type of cholesterol-lowering drug.
- Vitamin E, which can improve glucose tolerance in people with type 2 diabetes and may help to protect against coronary heart disease.
- Green tea which, when drunk regularly, can improve glucose control and reduce the risk of a heart attack.
- Pine Bark Extracts (known commercially as Pycnogenol®) which can also improve glucose control in type 2 diabetes, and help to protect against diabetic eye disease and unwanted blood clotting.
- The mineral selenium, which helps to improve glucose control and protect against coronary heart disease and cancer.

Information on each individual antioxidant follows to help you select those which are most suitable for you. Several supplements that combine antioxidants such as selenium and vitamins A, C and E are available. In addition to this you could also take alpha-lipoic acid, co-enzyme Q10 or Pycnogenol®, depending on whether you have diabetic polyneuropathy, retinopathy or high blood pressure, for example. If you wish to take several antioxidants together it is best to seek advice from a nutritional therapist.

Alpha-lipoic acid

What it is

Alpha-lipoic acid (also known as thioctic acid) is a vitamin-like substance that can be made in the body in small amounts. It works together with B group vitamins to speed metabolic reactions involved in energy production in cells. It is a powerful antioxidant and also regenerates other important antioxidants such as vitamins C and E, enhancing their effectiveness.

How it can help you

Alpha-lipoic acid is mainly used to boost energy levels, and combat chronic fatigue. It is also taken to help treat symptoms linked with nerve damage such as tingling, numbness or discomfort, and liver problems such as hepatitis and cirrhosis.

In a study involving 107 people with diabetes, those taking alpha-lipoic acid as an antioxidant (600mg/day for more than three months) had significantly lower levels of harmful oxidation reactions than those not taking it, even if they had poor glucose control and protein in their urine.[22]

Aiding glucose control Alpha-lipoic acid improves glucose control by increasing its removal from the blood circulation and its uptake into skeletal muscle cells by up to 50 per cent.[23] It is believed to both stimulate insulin activity and reduce insulin resistance, and has been shown to improve insulin sensitivity in people with type 2 diabetes.[24]

Reducing effects of diabetic neuropathy Alpha-lipoic acid is thought to reduce damage from oxidation to the fatty myelin sheath that surrounds our nerves,[25] and has been shown to improve the conduction of nerve signals and associated blood flow through small blood vessels in people with diabetic neuropathy (see page 27).[26]

In a study involving 120 people with diabetic polyneuropathy (which affects a number of nerves), it significantly reduced shooting and burning pain, numbness and prickling sensations.[27] Another trial involved 328 people with type 2 diabetes, who were given daily doses of alpha-lipoic acid for three weeks.[28] Their symptoms were reduced by 58 per cent on the higher dose (1200mg), 63 per cent on the middle dose (600mg) and 43 per cent on the lower dose (100mg), compared with a 38 per cent improvement in those taking a placebo. In a study involving 24 people with type 2 diabetes and polyneuropathy, those taking 600mg of ALA three times a day for three weeks experienced significant improvements in symptoms such as pain, burning, pins and needles and numbness in the feet, compared with those taking a placebo.[29]

By 1999, at least 15 clinical trials had been completed in Germany, along with those showing benefit in polyneuropathy and nerve conduction on doses of at least 600mg per day.[30]

Preventing kidney damage Damage from free radicals plays a major role in kidney damage in people with diabetes. Several studies have suggested that taking alpha-lipoic acid can reduce damage from oxidation and albumin in the urine (a sign of kidney leakage and damage) in people with diabetes, and reduce deterioration in kidney function.[31]

Where you find it

Carrots, yams, sweet potatoes, beets and red meat are all good sources. It is also made in small amounts within the body.

How much you need

A typical dose is 50 to 100mg daily as a general antioxidant, although higher doses of 600mg one to three times a day may be suggested for therapeutic use in people with diabetes who have polyneuropathy or kidney damage.

Side effects/safety

Mild skin rashes or gastrointestinal side effects have occurred, but such side effects have been rare.

Talk to your doctor before taking alpha-lipoic acid if you have heart, liver or kidney problems. Monitor blood glucose levels carefully when taking it, as it can stimulate uptake of glucose into muscle cells.

Vitamin A and carotenoids

What it is

Vitamin A is a fat-soluble vitamin that can be stored in the liver. Pre-formed vitamin A (retinol) is found only in animal foods, but some carotenoid plant pigments, such as betacarotene, can be converted into vitamin A in the body. Nutritionally, 6mcg of beta-carotene can provide around 1mcg of retinol. If your liver is in good shape, you convert, on average, around half the betacarotene you eat into vitamin A.

How it can help you

Vitamin A is a powerful antioxidant that also regulates genes involved in normal growth, development, healing and immunity. And, as anyone exhorted to eat carrots in their childhood knows, it's also essential for eyesight. In the eye, vitamin A is converted into a pigment in the retina, 'visual purple' (rhodopsin), which is essential for vision.

Improving insulin sensitivity Vitamin A does more than help us see and balance our genetic activity. It also helps to reduce insulin resistance in people with type 2 diabetes and metabolic syndrome. People with type 2 diabetes who obtain the most vitamin A from their diet are therefore the most efficient users of insulin.[32]

In Japan, a study[33] investigating the relationship between raised blood glucose levels, carotenoids and intake of fruit and vegetables among 288 people with either diabetes or glucose intolerance found that those with the highest intake of carrots and pumpkins (which are rich in carotenoids) were half as likely to have poor glucose tolerance as those with low intakes. Blood levels of the carotenoids alpha- and beta-carotenes, lycopene, beta-cryptoxanthin, zeaxanthin and lutein all showed a beneficial effect, which suggests that carotenoid-rich vegetables and fruits might protect against developing raised blood glucose levels.

A beneficial link between the metabolism of glucose and eating carotenoids from fruit and vegetables has also been shown in men at high risk of type 2 diabetes.[34]

Boosting artery health Research[35] on children with type 1 diabetes has shown that those with poor glucose control were more likely to lack antioxidant vitamin A and to have a higher risk of developing hardening and furring up of the arteries than those with good control. The researchers suggested that taking vitamin A supplements might help to protect the circulation of children with type 1 diabetes.

Improving vision Age-related macular degeneration (AMD) is the most common cause of registered blindness in people over 50. It is due to deterioration of the part of the retina that's involved in fine vision such as reading and recognising faces. The cause is unknown, but people who smoke, and have high blood pressure, elevated cholesterol levels and diabetes are at greatest risk.

The macula of the eye contains two carotenoid pigments, lutein and zeaxanthin (which can be made from lutein). Researchers have found that people with macular degeneration have, on average, 70 per cent less lutein and zeaxanthin in their eyes than those with healthy vision; poor dietary intake is thought to cause the breakdown of this vital part of the retina. Lutein helps to protect this delicate structure in the eye partly through its powerful antioxidant action, which neutralises harmful free radicals generated during the chemical processes involved in the detection of light. Lutein also helps to filter out visible blue light, which can cause photo-damage in the eye. This is why lutein and other carotenoids are sometimes referred to as 'nature's sunglasses'.[36,37]

People with the highest lutein and zeaxanthin levels in the retina have an 82 per cent lower risk of age-related macular degeneration than those with the lowest levels.[38] Getting adequate amounts of lutein is also linked to a significantly reduced risk of cataracts.[39]

A study involving almost 77,500 female nurses aged between 45 and 71 found that, after age, smoking, and other potential cataract risk factors were accounted for, those with the highest intake of lutein and zeaxanthin were 22 per cent less likely to develop cataracts severe enough to require extraction.[40]

Where you find it

Carotenoids are pigments found in dark green, leafy vegetables such as spinach, and yellow, orange or red fruits and vegetables, including carrots, sweetcorn, yams, apricots, mangoes and tomatoes. The carotenoid lutein is also present in egg yolk, giving it its yellow or orange colour.

Vitamin A (retinol) is found in animal foods such as liver, meats, oily fish, eggs, dairy products, butter, and margarine fortified by law to contain as much vitamin A as butter.

Vitamin A is easily destroyed by exposure to light, while beta-carotene is destroyed by heat and overcooking.

How much you need

The RDA for vitamin A is 800mcg. Ideally, you need around 6mcg mixed carotenoids daily.

Labels may give amounts of vitamin A in international units (IU); 1 IU of vitamin A is equivalent to 0.3mcg retinol, while 1mcg vitamin A = 3.33 IU.

Side effects/safety

Because vitamin A readily enters your nervous system, taking too much can cause symptoms of retinol poisoning – headache, irritability, blurred vision, nausea, weakness and fatigue. In the long term, excess vitamin A may increase the risk of liver cirrhosis.

Big doses of vitamin A (3000mcg daily or more) during pregnancy are associated with certain birth defects. Pregnant women should avoid taking supplements containing pre-formed retinol and should not eat liver or liver products. As vitamin A is vital for normal, healthy development in the womb, however, supplements aimed at pregnant women usually contain carotenoids such as betacarotene that can be converted into retinol when needed.

You should aim to limit your intake of vitamin A to less than 1500mcg per day. Do not combine supplements providing vitamin A (such as a multivitamin plus cod liver oil) without checking that you're not exceeding recommended levels.

Supplemental forms of betacarotene are best avoided by those who smoke. One trial found that people with a high risk of lung cancer from smoking did not benefit from taking betacarotene supplements; their risks of developing this cancer may even have risen. This was probably because the people involved were heavy smokers who may already have had early, undiagnosed lung cancer at the start of the trial, but this is another situation where it's best to err on the side of caution.

Excess carotenoids can cause a yellow-orange discolouration of skin. It may look like a cheap fake tan, but it isn't harmful and it resolves when you reduce the amount you take.

Vitamin C

What it is

Vitamin C – otherwise known as ascorbic acid – is a water-soluble vitamin that cannot be stored in the body in appreciable amounts. It's the main antioxidant found in body fluids. It protects cells from free radical damage, and also acts as an essential co-factor for at least 300 metabolic reactions. It is vital for the synthesis of collagen, a major structural protein in the body, making it necessary for the proper growth and repair of tissues.

How it can help you

Aiding glucose control Vitamin C is similar in structure to glucose and plays a role in glucose control and insulin action.[41,42,43] People with vitamin C deficiency can have abnormal blood glucose control similar to that seen in diabetes; correcting the deficiency returns their glucose balance to normal, although the exact mechanism is uncertain.[44] Vitamin C is less able to enter cells when blood glucose levels are raised, and this may result in what has been described as a 'localised scurvy' in people with diabetes. In fact, as blood vessel changes resulting from scurvy resemble those seen in people with diabetes, this localised lack of vitamin C may contribute to the blood vessel damage that occurs in diabetes.

Reducing glycosylation Interactions between protein and glucose, known as glycosylation, lead to tissue damage and premature ageing in people with diabetes. Vitamin C can significantly reduce the glycosylation of proteins. Taking 1g a day can reduce glycosylation of haemoglobin in the blood by 18 per cent, and albumin by 33 per cent after three months.[45] It's important to note that this effect, while beneficial, does affect blood tests to assess levels of HbA1c (see page 48), so if you take that test and are also supplementing vitamin C, you need to tell your doctor.

Reducing sorbitol formation When glucose levels are raised, some glucose is converted inside cells to a substance called sorbitol. While safe as a dietary sweetener, sorbitol is harmful when formed inside cells. If it builds up in cells, sorbitol can contribute to diabetic complications, especially those affecting the eyes (retinopathy, cataracts) and nervous system (peripheral neuropathy, which affects nerves other than those in the brain and spinal column).

Vitamin C has been shown to reduce sorbitol formation by blocking an enzyme crucial to the process. In one study,[46] taking 1g vitamin C per day for just two weeks reduced the amount of sorbitol within red blood cells by over 12 per cent, while in another study, taking 2g vitamin C daily reduced the build-up of sorbitol in red blood cells by 44.5 per cent in people with diabetes.[47] The researchers in the second study concluded that moderate supplementation with vitamin C might provide a 'simple, safe and effective means of preventing and ameliorating chronic complications of diabetes'.

A later study[48] found that taking even smaller amounts of vitamin C (100 or 600mg daily) could normalise red blood cell sorbitol levels in people with diabetes within 30 days, and that this reduction was not affected by how well the person was managing their diabetes.

Reducing cholesterol levels As an antioxidant, vitamin C protects cholesterol in the bloodstream from oxidation. So, as only oxidised cholesterol is linked with hardening and furring up of the arteries, vitamin C has the potential to help protect against heart attack and possibly stroke.

A significantly lower level of vitamin C has been found in the blood and white blood cells of people with diabetes who also have high cholesterol levels. People taking 500mg per day for 12 months[49] significantly lowered their cholesterol levels. This regime was also associated with a moderate fall in triglyceride levels, while blood fat levels in the control group, who were not taking vitamin C, remained the same. The researchers think vitamin C may help improve the liver's ability to flush cholesterol from the body.

In a placebo-controlled trial of 40 people with type 2 diabetes who also had raised cholesterol levels, 1g of vitamin C was taken daily for four months. The people taking vitamin C had improved glucose tolerance, lowered total and LDL cholesterol levels and less free radical damage. The percentage increase in the amount of vitamin C present in the fluid part of the blood (the plasma) was directly related to the fall in the percentage of LDL cholesterol, and the researchers concluded that vitamin C has an important role to play in managing type 2 diabetes.[50] Similar improvements in glucose control and cholesterol have been shown in other studies.[51]

Lowering risk of coronary heart disease A lack of vitamin C appears to be a risk factor for developing a heart attack or stroke. In one study involving over 6600 men and women, those with the highest vitamin C levels enjoyed a 27 per cent lower risk of coronary heart disease and a 26 per cent lower risk of stroke than those with low levels. The researchers concluded that these results could indicate that taking more vitamin C may decrease the risk of coronary heart disease and stroke.[52]

Vitamin C may also play a role in preventing symptoms in those with existing coronary artery disease,[53] and low levels are linked with an increased risk of developing angina.[54] A 10-year study involving 11,000 people has shown that men with the highest intakes of vitamin C have a 40 per cent lower risk of developing coronary heart disease and a 35 per cent lower risk of dying from it. For women taking the highest levels of vitamin C, there was a 25 per cent lower risk of coronary heart disease; they were also up to 42 per cent less likely to die from cancer. According to another study of 1605 middle-aged men, those who had vitamin C deficiency were 3.5 times more at risk of a heart attack than men with normal blood fluid (plasma) levels of vitamin C.[55]

A recent study involving over 19,000 adults aged 45 to 79 years found that circulating levels of vitamin C were inversely related to death from all causes over the four years of the study.[56] Researchers have also found that in elderly patients, taking low amounts of vitamin C was a strong predictor for risk of death by stroke.[57]

Improving dilation of blood vessels Vitamin C can improve blood flow and the dilation of blood vessels in people with diabetes.[58] This is an important finding because people with diabetes often have impaired blood flow, probably partly as a result of free radical damage as well as the inactivation of the body mechanism that dilates blood vessels.[59] Vitamin C may ease blood flow by acting on the 'signalling' molecule nitric oxide, much like Viagra. (Whether or not vitamin C supplements are helpful for men with diabetes who have erectile dysfunction remains to be seen.)

Preventing cataracts As I have mentioned, people with diabetes are more prone to cataracts because free radical damage can cloud proteins in the lens of the eye. Vitamin C is an important antioxidant in the eye: the level of this vitamin in your lens is 60 times higher than that found in your circulation. And its presence guards against cataract.

A study of 1380 people attending an ophthalmology outpatient clinic found that the people taking multivitamin and antioxidant supplements regularly had a 37 per cent lower risk of developing cataracts, and that dietary intakes of vitamin C, among other nutrients, decreased the risk.[60] Another study found that people taking 300mg vitamin C daily were 70 per cent less likely to develop cataracts than similar patients not taking supplements.[61]

The Nurses' Health Study found that 60 per cent of early cataracts occurred in relatively young women who had not taken vitamin C supplements; women who had taken vitamin C for at least 10 years had a 45 per cent decreased risk of developing cataracts as those who had not taken it.[62] Interestingly, those not taking vitamin C supplements still had a naturally high dietary intake of vitamin C, averaging 130mg – which is twice as high as the RDA – yet only those taking additional vitamin C seemed to obtain a benefit.

These findings were confirmed recently when women who took vitamin C supplements for at least 10 years were found to have a 77 per cent lower risk of developing early cataracts, and an 83 per cent lower risk of moderate cataracts, compared with women who did not use vitamin C. These studies suggest that long-term consumption of vitamin C supplements may substantially reduce the development of age-related cataracts[63] – so if you have diabetes, this is a very important finding.

Where you find it

Vitamin C is mainly found in fruit and vegetables, including berries, guavas, kiwis, citrus fruit, mangoes, green peppers and green sprouting vegetables such as broccoli, sprouts and watercress. Animal sources include kidney and liver.

Vitamin C is one of the most unstable vitamins, and up to two-thirds is lost by processing, prolonged cooking and storage.

How much you need

The new RDA for vitamin C is 80mg, although this is widely thought to be too low. A review of the vitamin in the *American Journal of Clinical Nutrition* recommended an intake of 90 to 100mg, minimum, for the optimum reduction of chronic disease risk in people without diabetes.[64] In the US, an expert scientific panel recently suggested that the average need of half the healthy individuals in a population might be 100mg a day of vitamin C, with a safety margin (to account for people who might need more) giving a proposed increased RDA of 120mg/day.[65]

For people without diabetes, the general consensus is that 120 to 250mg vitamin C is a good basic intake. Most studies have found that people with diabetes have at least 30 per cent lower circulating levels of vitamin C compared to those without diabetes.[66] This is due partly to the higher production of free radicals, and partly because lower levels of insulin means less vitamin C gets into cells.[67] Lack of vitamin C inside the cells can, in turn, lead to a number of problems, including an increased capillary leakiness, poor wound healing, raised cholesterol levels and reduced immunity. All this suggests that higher doses of 500mg to 1g vitamin C daily, or even more, have been suggested for people with diabetes. Taking 2 to 3g a day, in divided doses, does not appear to be harmful.

Side effects/safety

There has been a great deal of research into the safety of supplementing vitamin C. Claims that large doses trigger kidney stones have proved unfounded. However, if you have been repeatedly troubled by kidney stones or have kidney failure, or if you have inherited a defect in ascorbic acid or oxalate metabolism, you may be advised to restrict your daily vitamin C intake to approximately 100mg.

If you take 3g or more a day, you may find this causes indigestion or diarrhoea. This will settle when you reduce your dose, or take a buffered, non-acidic form of the vitamin such as Ester-C®. Interestingly, when you are ill, your vitamin C needs seem to increase to such an extent that you become much more tolerant of high doses and can take higher amounts before developing loose bowel motions.

As we've seen, the structure of vitamin C is similar to that of glucose. So if you're taking high doses of vitamin C and need to have a urine, blood or stool test, inform your doctor, as it can affect laboratory results (for HbA1c and urinary glucose, for instance).

Individuals with iron-storage disease such as haemochromatosis should not take vitamin C supplements except under medical advice, as it enhances the absorption of inorganic iron.

If you decide to take very high dose supplements and then decide to stop, you should reduce your intake slowly over a few weeks rather than suddenly cutting it off.

Co-enzyme Q10

What it is

Co-enzyme Q10 or CoQ10 is a vitamin-like substance also known as ubiquinone. It is needed to process oxygen in cells, and to generate energy-rich molecules. It also acts together with vitamin E to form a powerful antioxidant defence against atherosclerosis and heart disease.

Levels of CoQ10 start to decrease once you reach the age of 20, as dietary CoQ10 is absorbed less efficiently from the intestines and its production in body cells starts to fall. If you lack CoQ10, your cells – including those in the heart muscle – do not receive all the energy they need, so they function at a sub-optimal level and are more likely to become diseased and to age prematurely.

How it can help you

Improving glucose control It has been suggested that CoQ10 may increase insulin secretion by improving energy production within beta cells. This might explain why CoQ10 often improves beta cell function and glucose control in people with type 2 diabetes.[68]

Reducing blood stickiness CoQ10 seems to reduce the size and stickiness of platelets – blood fragments involved in clotting – and may also help to reduce the risk of blood clots that play a role in heart attack. In one study, volunteers taking 100mg of CoQ10 twice a day for 20 days were found to have significant reductions in platelet activity and platelet size.[69]

Improving blood vessel function Arterial disease is one of the main complications in people with type 2 diabetes. One study[70] found that the brachial (arm) artery in 40 people with type 2 showed impaired dilation, compared with those of non-diabetics. When some were given 200mg CoQ10 for 12 weeks, dilation in their brachial artery increased by 1.6 per cent, whereas those given a placebo experienced further deterioration in the artery. This improvement was not due to its antioxidant action. It's possible that it works via nitric oxide – like Viagra and vitamin C. CoQ10 may therefore be helpful for men with diabetes who also have problems achieving an erection.

Alleviating heart problems It has been shown that 50 to 75 per cent of people with various forms of heart disease are deficient in CoQ10. At least one study has found that the more severe the heart disease, the lower the levels of CoQ10. CoQ10 has therefore been used by some doctors to help treat coronary heart disease and congestive heart failure. It also seems to have a beneficial effect in reducing abnormal heart rhythms.[71]

When 22 people with heart failure were given 100mg of CoQ10, or a placebo, twice a day for 12 weeks, those taking CoQ10 showed significant improvements in how well their left ventricle (the lower left chamber of the heart) worked.[72] A trial involving 641 patients with congestive heart failure found that those taking 2mg per kg body weight CoQ10 a day for a year were admitted to hospital for treatment of complications significantly fewer times than those taking a placebo.[73]

In another trial, 424 patients with various forms of heart disease added CoQ10 to their usual drug regimes at doses of 75 to 600mg a day. After monitoring for an average of 17.8 months, 87 per cent showed significant improvements in heart function, with 43 per cent able to stop taking between one and three heart drugs.[74]

Reducing high blood pressure CoQ10 is thought to reduce high blood pressure by improving the elasticity and reactivity of the blood vessel wall. In a trial involving 18 people with 'essential' hypertension, where the cause is unknown, taking 100mg of CoQ10 a day significantly reduced blood pressure when compared with a placebo.[75] In another trial involving 109 people with essential hypertension, an average daily dose of 225mg CoQ10 was added in to their existing drug regime.[76] They experienced a significant, gradual improvement in blood pressure control and, overall, more than half the participants were able to stop taking between one and three antihypertensive drugs within a few months of starting CoQ10. Those receiving echocardiograms showed a significant improvement in the thickness and function of their left ventricle, making the heart's pumping action more efficient.

In a trial involving 74 people with type 2 diabetes and abnormal cholesterol levels, the participants received either 100mg of CoQ10 twice a day, 200mg fenofibrate each morning, both, or neither for

12 weeks.[77] The results showed that CoQ10 supplements improved both blood pressure and glucose control, although this did not seem to be due to its antioxidant effect – suggesting that other mechanisms (such as more flexible artery walls) may be involved.

Reducing the side effects of statin drugs People taking statin drugs to lower cholesterol levels (see page 65) reduce the production of CoQ10 in their body because these drugs block an enzyme (HMG-CoA) involved in CoQ10 manufacture.[78] In some cases, low CoQ10 levels in people with type 2 diabetes can cause diabetic cardiomyopathy, a condition that can lead to congestive heart failure. This is reversible if you take CoQ10 supplements. So, if you have diabetes or metabolic syndrome and need cholesterol-lowering drugs, you will benefit by taking a CoQ10 supplement.

Where you find it

Dietary sources of CoQ10 include meat, fish, wholegrains, nuts and green vegetables.

How much you need

There is no accepted recommended daily amount, and average intakes are estimated at 3 to 5mg a day for meat eaters and 1mg a day for vegetarians. Supplements range from 10 to 200mg, meant to be taken daily. Higher amounts of 600mg a day may be taken for therapeutic use. CoQ10 is best taken with food to improve absorption, as it is fat-soluble. It usually takes at least three weeks and occasionally up to three months before the full beneficial effects are noticed.

Side effects/safety

No serious side effects have been reported, even at high doses – only occasional mild nausea.

Vitamin E

What it is

Vitamin E is actually a group of eight fat-soluble vitamins, of which the most active form is d-alpha-tocopherol. It provides the main antioxidant protection for body fats, including cell membranes, has a strengthening effect on muscle fibres and improves skin suppleness and healing. It also plays an important role in immune function. Vitamin E and selenium (see page 147) work synergistically – that is, better together than the sum of each – in the formation of antibodies in the immune system. Both have been found to increase antibody synthesis thirtyfold, as well as improving the body's response to influenza vaccinations. Vitamin C is needed to regenerate vitamin E when it has carried out its antioxidant function.

How it can help you

Lowering blood fats People with diabetes who took 1200IU (800mg) natural vitamin E for eight weeks had significantly reduced oxidation of circulating LDL cholesterol than those not taking supplements.[79] In another study, taking a modest amount of vitamin E (100IU or 67mg daily) was shown to lower levels of free radicals in blood fats as well as levels of the triglyceride levels themselves.[80]

Improving glucose tolerance Some studies have shown that vitamin E improves glucose tolerance in people with type 2 diabetes,[81,82,83] although it may take three months or more for the benefits to become apparent. In one study, taking 1350IU (900mg) vitamin E every day for four months lowered free radical production and improved insulin action in people with type 2 diabetes, compared with people who did not supplement with it.[84]

Another study came up with a finding that was, perhaps, even more important. Researchers found that a low intake of vitamin E was a significant risk factor for the development of type 2 diabetes. When 944 men without diabetes and aged 42 to 60 were followed for four years, those with below-average intakes of vitamin E were almost four times more likely to have an abnormal blood glucose tolerance test or to have developed type 2 diabetes than those with above-average intakes.[85]

When people with type 2 diabetes received 1350IU of vitamin E a day for four months, they showed improved glucose tolerance and insulin sensitivity. However, when 36 people with type 2 diabetes were given lower doses of either 400IU (268mg) or 800IU (536mg) of vitamin E daily, no significant effects were seen until after six months of treatment, and no effect was noted in the group receiving the lowest dose.[86] This, and other studies,[87] suggest that a dose of at least 800IU is needed in people with diabetes to produce improvements in glucose control.

Reducing glycosylation Like vitamin C, vitamin E also seems to reduce glycosylation of proteins,[88,89] – a significant factor in premature ageing – although not all studies have confirmed this,[90] and higher doses (above 800IU per day) do seem to be needed. When 1340IU (around 900mg) of vitamin E was given to 25 elderly type 2 diabetics for three months, their levels of glycosylated haemoglobin fell by 9 per cent, and their 'fasting' glucose by 10 per cent. Their total cholesterol levels were also reduced.[91]

Protecting against coronary heart disease Vitamin E's antioxidant prowess focuses on fats, and that includes blood fats. In addition to its role neutralising free radicals, it also reduces platelet clumping and so thins the blood, and has an anti-inflammatory effect.[92,93] These properties are thought to slow hardening and furring up of the arteries, and reduce the risk of fatty plaques in the coronary arteries rupturing and triggering coronary thrombosis – the formation of harmful blood clots.

In middle-aged European males 40 to 59 years old, it has been shown that low blood levels of vitamin E are linked to a higher incidence of death, at any age, from coronary artery disease – in which the arteries are so furred up with plaques that the heart fails to receive enough oxygen.[94] Some large studies show a 40 per cent reduction in coronary heart disease rates in both men and women taking vitamin E supplements – the risk is lowest in those taking 100IU (around 67mg) vitamin E per day for at least two years.[95,96]

These findings are not isolated. Vitamin E gained widespread medical acceptance when the Cambridge Heart Antioxidant Study

(CHAOS) was published in 1996.[97] Just over 2000 patients with coronary heart disease were divided into two groups. Half took vitamin E for 18 months, half received a placebo. Taking high doses of vitamin E (at least 400IU daily) was found to reduce the risk of a heart attack by 77 per cent. Not only was the difference highly statistically significant: amazingly, it seemed that the group treated with vitamin E were at no greater risk of a heart attack than people without coronary heart disease. As a result, many physicians now recommend high doses of vitamin E for older people, especially those at risk of a heart attack.

Improving brain function The solid part of the brain is quite fatty, so vitamin E plays a significant protective role in it, fending off oxidation of brain cells. This makes for a healthier brain and boosts our cognition, or thinking skills. Thus high levels of vitamin E are strongly associated with better cognitive scores, compared with those having the lowest vitamin E intakes.[98]

Protecting against cataracts Vitamin E also helps to protect against cataracts which, as we've seen, are a significant risk in people with diabetes. In one study, people with the highest intake of vitamin E were found to be half as likely to develop cataracts severe enough to need surgery, compared to those with the lowest intakes.[99] A study of 1380 people attending an ophthalmology outpatient clinic found that regular use of multivitamin and antioxidant supplements, combined with foods rich in vitamin E among other nutrients, decreased the risk of developing cataracts by 37 per cent.[100]

Where you find it

The richest sources of vitamin E are wheatgerm oil, avocados, butter and margarine, wholemeal cereals, nuts and seeds, oily fish, eggs and broccoli. Fresh raw foods and supplements are the best sources. Processing and exposure to air rapidly deplete the vitamin. Even freezing causes it to leach away: frozen foods can lose up to 70 per cent of their vitamin E content within 14 days.

The vitamin E content of foods and supplements is usually expressed in terms of alpha-tocopherol equivalents. Synthetic alpha-tocopherol (dl-alpha tocopherol) has less biological strength than natural-source vitamin E (d-alpha tocopherol), so if you're supplementing go for the stronger natural type.

Sometimes the amount of vitamin E is expressed in IU rather than milligrams; 1IU = 0.67mg alpha-tocopherol equivalents or, conversely, 1mg = 1.5IU.

How much you need

The EU RDA for vitamin E is 12mg, but generally speaking, the more polyunsaturated fats you eat, the more vitamin E you need. Doses of up to 540mg (800IU) a day or more may be taken over the long term with no apparent ill effects, although an upper limit of 1g a day is usually suggested.

High-dose vitamin E is best taken together with other antioxidants, such as vitamin C, mixed carotenoids and selenium. There is evidence to support that many antioxidants work synergistically – better together than individually. This is especially true of vitamin E, which constantly needs to be regenerated back to its active form by other antioxidants such as vitamin C.

Side effects/safety

High intakes of vitamin E can cause headache, fatigue, gastro-intestinal distress, double vision and muscle weakness, but this only usually occurs above amounts of 3000mg a day.

Tea and green tea extracts
....

What it is

Not every wildly popular food or drink is good for us. So it's lucky that tea is such a rich source of antioxidants.

Two main varieties are used, the smaller-leaved China tea (*C. sinensis sinensis*) and the larger-leaved Assam tea (*C. sinensis assamica*). Green tea is unfermented, black tea fermented, and 'brown' or oolong tea is somewhere in between. White tea is similar to green tea but only made from new tea buds, picked before they open. It has the lowest levels of caffeine.

As we have seen, tea has abundant antioxidant polyphenols such as catechin and epicatechin, which together have an antioxidant action at least 100 times more powerful than that of vitamin C, and 25 times more powerful than vitamin E. Green tea antioxidants are converted into less active antioxidants such as theaflavins and thearubigins during fermentation. Despite this, drinking four to five cups of black tea a day will still provide over half your dietary needs for flavonoid antioxidants – other sources include fruit and vegetables, especially apples and onions. Tea is also a rich source of phytochemicals and the trace element manganese, and is one of the few natural sources of fluoride which helps to protect against tooth decay.

How it can help you

Improving glucose control Green tea antioxidants (catechins) appear to have an insulin-like action.[101] They can improve glucose and fat metabolism, enhance insulin sensitivity, and promote fat burning rather than fat storage – especially around the abdomen – which may make it helpful for people with metabolic syndrome or type 2 diabetes. When 20 people with type 2 diabetes drank 1.5 litres oolong tea every day for 30 days, their blood glucose levels fell by 30 per cent compared with a regime substituting water for the tea. The researchers concluded that oolong tea may be an effective addition to other treatments for type 2 diabetes.[102]

Black tea has been shown to have anti-diabetes effects similar to those of green tea.[103]

Protecting against coronary heart disease Drinking either black, green or white tea has beneficial effects on blood fats, blood pressure and blood stickiness, and can decrease the risk of coronary heart disease and stroke.

In one study, out of a group of 3430 men and women 30 to 70 years old, those who drank more than six cups of black tea a day had a significantly lower risk of developing coronary heart disease than non-tea drinkers, even when other factors such as smoking, weight, family history, fat intake, blood levels and diabetes were taken into account.[104] Another study found that drinking just one cup of tea a day almost halved the risk of having a heart attack compared with people who drank no tea.[105] Other studies have put the number of cups for this level of protection at four. The effect is thought to come from tea's antioxidant action, which reduces the oxidation of LDL cholesterol, so less is deposited in artery walls.

In Japan, 512 men and women undergoing testing for arterial damage were asked about the amount of green tea they drank.[106] Those who drank more tended to have a lower risk of coronary artery disease in men, but not in women. In a sub-group of men who did not have diabetes, those drinking 2 to 3 cups of green tea per day were half as likely to have significant narrowing of the coronary arteries, and those drinking 4 or more cups per day were 60 per cent less likely to be affected. These results indicate that green tea may be protective against coronary atherosclerosis (hardening and furring of the arteries), at least in men who do not have diabetes.

Aiding weight loss An extract from green tea has been shown to boost the body's calorie-burning rate by as much as 40 per cent over a 24-hour period. Clinical trials involving 80 overweight men and women who took green tea extracts found they lost 3.5kg over three months, with a decrease in waist circumference of 1cm.

Protection against infections Green, black and oolong tea have antibacterial[107] and antiviral[108] actions to help boost immunity to infections. A high intake – possibly greater than that obtained by most tea drinkers – may be needed to obtain these benefits, however.[109]

How much you need

Drinking at least four to five cups of tea per day appears to be most beneficial. Green tea extracts are also available in supplement form.

Side effects/safety

No significant health problems have been linked with drinking tea.

Pine bark extracts

What it is

Extracts from the bark of the French maritime pine (known commercially as Pycnogenol®) contain a rich blend of natural fruit acids and antioxidants known as proanthocyanidins. Research suggests the antioxidant action of Pycnogenol® is over 100 times more powerful than vitamin E and vitamin C and 16 times more active than grapeseed extracts.[110] As Pycnogenol® enhances the effects of other antioxidants such as CoQ10 and vitamins C and E, they are often combined in supplements.

Pine bark extracts have a beneficial effect on the circulation, reducing hardening and furring up of the arteries, and thinning the blood by lessening platelet clumping. As a result they also reduce the risk of coronary heart disease and stroke. These extracts are widely taken to treat conditions associated with poor circulation, including diabetes, and are helpful for treating impotence, varicose veins, thread veins, macular degeneration in the eye, peripheral vascular disease (see page 33), intermittent claudication (see page 34) and leg cramps. The extracts are also used as a substitute for aspirin taken to reduce the risk of deep vein thrombosis on long-haul flights.

How it can help you

Improved glucose control People with type 2 diabetes who take 50 to 200mg pine bark extracts have lower blood glucose levels and healthier blood vessels.[111] In a study involving 30 people, participants took increasing doses starting at 50mg for three weeks, then receiving 100mg, 200mg and 300mg, each for a three-week period. Fasting blood glucose levels fell significantly, depending on the size of the dose, until 200mg was reached, at which point they plateaued. HbA1c levels (see page 48) decreased, but insulin levels were not affected, which showed that the effect was not due to the stimulation of insulin secretion. A double-blind placebo-controlled study involving 77 people has confirmed that pine bark extracts do lower glucose levels.[112]

Protecting against eye disease In at least five clinical studies involving a total of 1289 people, Pycnogenol® has been shown to help seal leaky blood vessels in the eyes of people with diabetes.[113] All these studies showed that the extract reduced the progression of retinopathy (see page 24) and partially restored visual acuity, helping to preserve vision. In one study,[114] 40 people with diabetes, atherosclerosis and other vascular diseases involving the retina were given either placebo or 50mg of Pycnogenol® three times a day for two months. Those given the extract showed no deterioration in retinal function and, in fact, recovered some of their visual acuity, while in those receiving placebo, retinopathy progressively worsened during the trial and visual acuity significantly decreased. Ophthalmic tests showed that compared to the placebo, the extract boosted the circulation of blood within the retina and reduced leakage from the capillaries. It has been suggested that Pycnogenol® may bind to the blood vessel wall proteins to 'seal' leaking areas.

Protecting against blood clots Preliminary studies suggest pine bark extract is as effective as aspirin at reducing abnormal blood clotting in smokers. One German study found that 100mg Pycnogenol® prevented platelet clumping in 22 heavy smokers, while another found that 125mg Pycnogenol® was as effective as 500mg aspirin in preventing the increased blood pressure normally seen after smoking in 16 American smokers.[115] Other studies suggest that a dose of 200mg Pycnogenol® is more effective at reducing platelet clumping than lower doses. Aspirin significantly increases bleeding time (typically from 167 to 236 seconds) at therapeutic doses, while Pycnogenol® does not. These studies suggest Pycnogenol® is as effective in preventing increased susceptibility to clotting as aspirin, but without the side effects.

How much you need

The usual dose is 50 to 200mg daily.

Side effects/safety

No significant side effects from taking pine bark extract have been reported.

Selenium

What it is

Selenium is an essential trace element that acts as a co-factor in the action of many antioxidant enzymes. As a result, selenium helps to protect against a wide variety of degenerative diseases such as hardening and furring up of the arteries, cataracts, arthritis, stroke, heart attack and cancer. Selenium is essential for cell growth and immune function, and is also important for immunity.

Compared with non-diabetics, people with diabetes have significantly lower levels of selenium[116,117,118] – possibly because of a higher need for antioxidants, which would swiftly deplete dietary selenium. A study[119] designed to assess the effects of antioxidant status on blood stickiness in 20 people with type 1 diabetes found that selenium concentrations in red blood cells were markedly reduced in people with diabetes, compared to those in 20 people without diabetes, and that these low levels were associated with increased thickness of the blood, or viscosity. Selenium levels have also been found to be low in people with leg ulcers.[120] So if you have diabetes, supplementing selenium may well be a good idea.

How it can help you

Improving glucose control Selenium has been shown to have a number of insulin-like actions: it stimulates the uptake of glucose into muscle cells, and regulates metabolic pathways involving glucose and fatty acids.[121] The mechanisms are not precisely known, but it is thought that selenium activates proteins that tell the cells when insulin is present.

Protecting against coronary heart disease Although the results don't always agree, it has been found that the higher the level of selenium intake, the lower the incidence of coronary heart disease.[122] The most likely reason is that selenium has an anti-clotting effect on the interactions between platelets and cells lining the heart.[123]

Protecting against pancreatitis Some people with diabetes suffer from chronic pancreatitis, an inflammation of the pancreas. It's known that a deficiency in antioxidants, and especially of

147

selenium, also plays a role in the development of this painful condition. Supplementing with a combination of antioxidants, including selenium, may reduce the pain, the frequency of acute attacks and the need for surgery.[124]

Protecting against cancer Selenium is emerging as an important preventive of cancers. In a study involving over 1300 people, those receiving 200mcg selenium a day had a 52 per cent lower risk of death from cancer, and significant reductions in the incidences of lung, colorectal, prostate and total cancers compared with those receiving a placebo.[125]

A similar study looked at the effects of 200mcg selenium supplementation in 974 men with previous skin cancer also found significant reductions of 50 per cent in total cancer deaths. Prostate cancer incidence fell by 63 per cent, colorectal cancer incidence by 58, lung cancer by 46 per cent and liver cancer by 35 per cent. The blinded phase of the trial was therefore stopped early, as it was considered unethical to withhold selenium from those in the placebo groups.[126]

These findings were supported when toenail clippings were collected from over 33,700 men; those with the highest levels of selenium were found to be 65 per cent less likely to develop prostate cancer over a five-year period than those with low levels.[127] As new research from Canada suggests that people with diabetes may be twice as likely to develop pancreatic cancer, and three times more likely to develop liver cancer, optimising your selenium intake could be an excellent idea.

Where you find it

High-protein bread made from Canadian and American wheat has a high level of selenium. Because of changes in policy, most Europeans now eat bread made from varieties of wheat grown within the EC, which are low in selenium. As a result, there is widespread concern that a healthy diet can no longer provide adequate intakes of selenium in many parts of Europe.

Other food sources include Brazil nuts, seafood, offal, wholegrains, onions, garlic, broccoli, cabbage, mushrooms, radishes and celery.

How much you need

The newly set EU RDA for selenium is 55mcg a day. Between 1975 and 1994, selenium intakes almost halved in the UK, from 60 to 34mcg per day.[128] Given the sometimes spectacular benefits of taking it, it would seem a very good idea to supplement.

Side effects/safety

An upper safe level of 300mcg selenium daily has recently been suggested. Toxicity can occur with intakes above 800mcg a day, leading to a garlic odour on the breath, fragile or black fingernails, a metallic taste in the mouth, dizziness, nausea and hair loss.

9

The B Vitamins

Did your mother endlessly nag you to 'eat up your vegetables' when you were a child? She was so right. Take spinach: a vitamin powerhouse, it contains vitamins A and C and the B vitamin folic acid, not to mention important minerals. Cauliflower sports a whole range of Bs, while broccoli, peppers, carrots and the rest are bursting with a range of vital micronutrients. Together with fruits, they provide a nutritional cornucopia that is literally essential for life, keeping your body systems in top working order by:

• converting fats and carbohydrates into energy
• digesting foods
• promoting cell division and growth
• repairing damaged tissues
• keeping your blood healthy
• fighting infection
• promoting mental alertness
• encouraging healthy reproduction.

Vitamins

There are 13 major vitamins that either cannot be synthesised in the body, or are made in such tiny amounts that they fail to meet requirements – such as vitamin D and niacin. So you have to get them in your diet, or from supplements.

But this isn't a cut-and-dried process. As we've seen, one person's vitamin requirements will rarely match another's. And if you are diabetic, your needs for certain vitamins will be much greater.

Whatever your needs, if you fail to get enough, you'll know it. The saying 'you are what you eat' was never more true than for these important micronutrients. So you may start to experience symptoms such as:
- dry, itchy skin
- tiredness and lack of energy
- poor wound healing
- increased susceptibility to infection.

How quickly these problems develop will depend on how quickly your body's store of a particular vitamin runs out. In the case of folic acid, for example, symptoms of deficiency may show within weeks, as very little is stored in the body. In contrast, your body usually has good stores of vitamin B12, and a deficiency may take years to show up. In general, the more fat-soluble a vitamin, the better your body can store it. Vitamins are therefore divided into two main groups:
- the fat-soluble vitamins (A, D, E and K), which can dissolve in fat and are stored effectively in your body, mainly in your liver
- the water-soluble vitamins (B group and C), which dissolve in water, and are easily lost in your urine. These cannot be stored in appreciable amounts (with the exception of vitamin B12), and you must continually replenish them from your diet.

B vitamins

In Chapter 8 we explored the many ways the antioxidant vitamins A, C and E combat both diabetes and the range of serious health problems that can attend it. This chapter looks at the best of the rest – the B group vitamins. All the B group vitamins are beneficial for people with diabetes as they are involved in the processes which produce energy within body cells. As well as having a useful effect on glucose control, folic acid and vitamin B12 also help to protect against coronary heart disease and other circulatory problems. Some people may need more B vitamins depending on their general health.
- Some B vitamins, such as B2 (riboflavin), appear to help protect against cataracts.
- Vitamin B3 (niacin) and B6 may help to reduce the risk of a heart attack.

- B6 is especially helpful for those with peripheral arterial disease or neuropathy.

Supplements that supply B group vitamins, including folic acid, are widely available and as a minimum it is useful to take one supplying at least the recommended daily amount (RDA) of each.

But before we look at each of the B group vitamins in turn, we need to look at an amino acid – a building block of protein – that is closely linked both with diabetes, and a deficiency in the B group vitamins.

Villain of the piece: homocysteine

Homocysteine, an amino acid in the blood, is turning out to be a major culprit in a number of degenerative diseases.

When it builds up in the blood, homocysteine damages the lining of your artery walls so they become narrow and inelastic. A raised homocysteine level is now recognised as an independent risk factor for hardening and furring up of the arteries, coronary heart disease, stroke, peripheral vascular disease and other conditions associated with abnormal blood clotting.[129,130,131]

If your level of homocysteine increases by just 5mcg/l, your risk of coronary heart disease will increase by an alarming 20 to 30 per cent,[132] and it is estimated that as many as 10 per cent of cardiovascular disease cases are due to raised homocysteine levels.[133] A study in the US[134] detected raised homocysteine levels in 42 per cent of people with stroke, 28 per cent with peripheral vascular disease, and 30 per cent with coronary heart disease, making it as least as important a risk factor as abnormal cholesterol levels and smoking. It is thought to damage artery walls by generating free radicals,[135] and by activating blood clotting factors. A raised homocysteine level is also linked with a number of other serious medical conditions, including osteoporosis, Alzheimer's disease and birth defects.

All of this begs the question, How much is too much? Unfortunately, we're not yet entirely sure, as the minimum safe blood level of homocysteine is still uncertain. Initially, it was suggested as between 8 and 15micromol/l,[136] but some experts now feel that homocysteine levels above 6.9micromol/l may be harmful for your long-term health. Homocysteine levels naturally rise with age, however, and a level of 12micromol/l or under may be acceptable for those aged over 60.

Risk from homocysteine

Homocysteine Level	Risk Level
6.9micromol/l	Optimum (low risk)
7 – 9.9micromol/l	Mild risk
10 – 12.9micromol/l	Moderate risk
13 – 20micromol/l	High risk
Over 20micromol/l	Very high risk

If you have a personal or family history of coronary heart disease, or other risk factors for this disease, it is a good idea to have your homocysteine level checked. If this is not available on the NHS, via your GP, a self-administered pin-prick blood test is now available from some pharmacies, or can be ordered on-line at www.yorktest.com.

The homocysteine/diabetes link

Not only do homocysteine levels tend to rise with age; higher levels are also associated more closely with diabetes – but type 2 rather than type 1. When levels of the amino acid were measured in a group of 91 children with type 1 diabetes, for example, they were no different than those found in a similar group of children without diabetes.[137]

Metabolic syndrome and type 2 diabetes (both characterised by raised insulin levels) do seem to be associated with higher levels of homocysteine in some studies, although not all, which may be one of the factors responsible for the increased risk of cardiovascular complications in these conditions.[138,139,140] High levels of insulin are thought to affect homocysteine levels in a number of ways – possibly through effects on kidney filtration or by affecting the enzymes needed to break it down. It seems that the younger the onset of type 2 diabetes, and the poorer the glucose control, the most likely you are to develop a rapid increase in homocysteine levels.[141]

Risk factors for cardiovascular disease (heart attack, stroke) were assessed in a group of people with both a raised homocysteine level and type 2 diabetes, and compared with a similar group of people with type 2 diabetes but normal levels of homocysteine. The researchers found that, compared to people without diabetes, people with type 2 diabetes had significantly higher levels of blood clotting factors, whether or not they also had raised homocysteine levels. Those with both type 2 diabetes *and* high levels of homocysteine were then given high doses of folic acid (15mg daily) and vitamin B6 (600mg pyridoxine daily), which produced a significant fall in homocysteine levels from 12.3 to 9.1 micromol/l. The level of blood clotting factors did not change significantly, but as these are all independent risk factors for heart disease, this is not surprising.[142]

Peripheral vascular disease, in which the arteries that supply blood to the legs harden and fur up, is one of the potential complications of long-standing diabetes. A study of people with type 2 diabetes and peripheral vascular disease found that boosted levels of homocysteine were associated with more severe narrowing of the arteries.[143]

Another study linking peripheral vascular disease and improvements from consuming folate, or folic acid – one of the B vitamins – is not surprising, given the homocysteine connection. In a 12-year trial, it was found that for every 400mcg per day increase in the amount of dietary folic acid they consumed, the participants' risk of developing peripheral vascular disease was found to decrease by 21 per cent. Men with the highest folate intake (840mcg per day) were 33 per cent less likely to be affected than those with the lowest intakes (244mcg per day). Less strong associations were also found for intakes of vitamin B6 and B12. These results suggest that higher intakes of folate acid may help to prevent peripheral vascular disease.[144]

Homocysteine levels are also implicated in increased risk of developing nerve damage, or neuropathy, in people with type 2 diabetes. One study found that every rise of 5 micromol/l in homocysteine levels increased the risk of diabetic neuropathy by between two and threefold.[145] Raised homocysteine levels are also associated with an increased risk of developing kidney problems,[146,147] or nephropathy, and the eye condition retinopathy.[148] (See Chapter 2 for a discussion of these complications of diabetes.)

People with diabetes appear to be more susceptible to the harmful effects of homocysteine on the circulation. In a study of 231 people, 60 per cent of whom had type 2 diabetes, homocysteine levels above 12 micromol/l were associated with thickened walls in the carotid artery, which supplies blood to the head, but those with diabetes had a more pronounced thickening than those without.[149] One reason may be reduced levels of the protective body chemical S-adenosylmethionine or SAMe, which is found in red blood cells.

Higher levels of homocysteine have also been linked to a decline in mental function in later life, and this has been shown in studies with people who have both type 2 diabetes and raised homocysteine levels.[150]

The good news in all this is that if you're keeping your diabetes well in check, you are likely to be keeping your homocysteine levels under control, too. When 95 people with type 2 diabetes were followed for three years, those who improved their glucose control over that time (as shown by a fall in levels of glycosylated HbA1c) also lowered their homocysteine levels. By contrast, those whose glucose control worsened had higher levels of homocysteine.[151] Hearteningly, this study suggested that people with type 2 diabetes can see the benefits even when their improvements in glucose control are relatively modest.

How homocysteine levels can be lowered

The link between homocysteine and diabetes is a serious one, and it is becoming increasingly evident that if you have type 2 diabetes or metabolic syndrome in particular, you'll need to pay attention not just to glucose levels in the blood, but levels of homocysteine too. Luckily, lowering your levels of this amino acid couldn't be simpler. It's pretty much all down to a handful of B vitamins: B12, folate (also known as folic acid) and B6.

Although between 10 and 15 per cent of the general population (and almost 30 per cent of those with coronary heart disease) do not break down homocysteine as well as they should, taking enough folate seems to keep homocysteine levels down even in many of the people with this inherited abnormality. Generally speaking, the higher your intake of B12, B6 and folate, the lower your level of homocysteine.[152,153]

At the moment, staggering numbers of people are deficient in these vitamins, however. In the US, for instance, one survey suggests that only 40 to 50 per cent of people obtain enough folate from their diet to process homocysteine normally.

How much should one take for maximum effect? So far, the research has not led to any hard-and-fast rules.

One analysis[154] of 12 trials suggested that taking 0.5 to 5.7mg folic acid per day could reduce elevated homocysteine levels by 25 per cent, while adding 0.02 to 1mg of vitamin B12 a day lowered them a further 7 per cent.

In a study of 350 people aged 65 to 75 years, folic acid supplements of 400 to 600mcg per day were needed to produce significant lowering of homocysteine levels, compared to a placebo.[155] Because elderly people tend not to absorb as much of the vitamin, the researchers estimated that a total intake of 926mcg per day was needed to avoid folate deficiency and lower cardiovascular risk. The addition of B12 is doubly important here, as folate can mask early signs of vitamin B12 deficiency, which can lead to a form of spinal cord damage known as sub-acute combined degeneration.

As you can see, there is considerable leeway in the optimal amount of B vitamins to take to counter high homocysteine levels. But if you have had a homocysteine test, the following table shows suggestions for how much to supplement. Note that along with supplementation, you need to follow a healthy, vitamin-rich diet.

Suggested doses of B vitamins

Homocysteine Level Level micromol/l	Risk Level	Supplements
6.9 or below	Optimal	400mcg daily for women planning a baby
7 – 9.9	Mild	3mg B6, 100mcg B12, 400mcg folic acid

10 – 12.9	Moderate	10mg B6, 100mcg B12, 1mg folic acid
13 – 20	High	50mg B6, 500mcg B12, 2mg folic acid
Over 20	Very high	100mg B6, 1mg B12, 5mg folic acid

You can find guidelines for healthy eating in Chapter 5. While keeping in mind my caveats in that chapter regarding alcohol consumption, note that the occasional glass of beer could be beneficial in the context of homocysteine control. Beer has long been known to be a good source of B vitamins, and one study of 155 people with type 2 diabetes found that those who drank beer had higher vitamin B12 and folic acid levels, and lower homocysteine levels.[156] A genuine case of 'a little of what you fancy does you good'!

Homocysteine, metformin and the Bs

One of the main treatments for type 2 diabetes is a drug called metformin (see page 45). Recent evidence suggests that treatment with metformin for just four months was associated with a 7 per cent fall in folate levels, and a 14 per cent fall in vitamin B12 levels, which led to a 4 per cent increase in homocysteine levels. This finding needs further investigation, but if you take metformin, it's wise to ensure you have a good intake of these B group vitamins.[157]

Realistically speaking, however, you'll need to get most of your Bs from food, and supplements. The following pages give you the lowdown on each member of this valuable vitamin family.

Vitamin B1 (thiamin or thiamine)

What it is

Vitamin B1 is a water-soluble vitamin that is readily lost from the body. Most people only have enough stored to last one month, so a regular dietary supply is essential.

How it can help you

Vitamin B1 plays a central role in metabolism and in the way nerves and muscle cells conduct messages. It is involved in the production of energy from glucose, the function of beta cells and the regulation of glucose metabolism, and may be involved in the transport of glucose within cells.[158] It also helps to maintain feelings of calm, alertness and mental energy.

Preventing arterial disease One of the effects of high insulin and glucose levels in people with type 2 diabetes is that the smooth muscle cells lining their arteries tend to overgrow, which contributes to hardening and furring up of the arteries, or atherosclerosis. One study looked at people with type 2 diabetes who needed lower limb amputation due to severe atherosclerosis. Smooth muscle cells were taken from their artery linings and exposed to high levels of glucose and insulin in laboratory cultures; one group also had thiamin added to the culture fluid. The cells in the cultures without thiamin increased in number over a six-day period, as expected, but the cells not exposed to thiamin did not – suggesting that B1 could have an important role in delaying the onset of atherosclerosis in people with type 2.[159]

Preventing diabetic retinopathy German and American scientists have found that treating diabetic rats with high doses of benfotiamine, a lipid-soluble form of vitamin B1, helps to prevent diabetic retinopathy[160] – although these findings have yet to be investigated in humans.[161]

Alleviating diabetic neuropathy Vitamin B1 may help reduce the symptoms of tingling and numbness that can occur in diabetic neuropathy.

Where you find it

Dietary sources include unrefined wholegrains (although in the UK, white and brown flour are fortified with thiamin to replace losses during production), meat products (especially pork and duck), seafood, dairy products, eggs, yeast extract, pulses, fruit, nuts and vegetables. Thiamin is easily lost during food processing and cooking. For example, freezing meats reduces their thiamin content by up to 50 per cent, while cooking meat at 200°C lowers thiamin content by another 20 per cent.

How much you need

The new EU RDA for thiamin is 1.1mg. Older people need more B1, yet many people over the age of 55 don't get enough. For them, nutritional therapists may recommend 50 to 100mg per day. In general, the more carbohydrate you eat, the more thiamin you will need. A lack of thiamin may lead to glucose intolerance. Some studies have found that people with type 2 diabetes tend to have lower levels of B1 than people without diabetes.[162,163] People taking diuretics may lose enough thiamin in their urine to cause a deficiency.

Side effects/safety

Vitamin B1 is relatively non-toxic, as excess is easily lost through urination. High daily doses (100mg thiamin hydrochloride or more) may cause headache, nausea, irritability, insomnia, rapid pulse and weakness. These symptoms will stop once you cease taking the supplements.

Vitamin B2 (riboflavin)

What it is

Vitamin B2 is a water-soluble vitamin and as such, can't be stored in the body, so you will need to have a regular supply from diet or supplements. Some studies have found that people with type

2 diabetes tend to have lower blood levels of B2 compared with similar people who don't have diabetes.[164] One study found that children with type 1 diabetes were four times more likely to have a B2 deficiency.[165] Children with type 1 are also likely to have a deteriorated riboflavin metabolism, and excrete more B2 in the urine, the longer they have had diabetes.[166]

In one study, distinct alterations in the metabolism of B2 and less B2 within circulating red blood cells were found in 35 children with type 1 diabetes. The researchers suggested people with type 1 may excrete B2 in the urine at a faster rate than people without diabetes, which may mean they need to obtain more from their diet or from supplements.[167]

How it can help you

Vitamin B2 plays a crucial role in the production of energy and the metabolism of proteins, fats and carbohydrate in the body. It's thought to play a key role in the way the insulin-producing beta cells detect glucose. It has even been suggested that a lack of vitamin B2, or abnormalities in its metabolism, might be linked with the development of diabetes. Defects in riboflavin metabolism appear to be 'far from uncommon' in contributing to the development of type 2 diabetes.[168]

Preventing cataracts B2 appears to play an essential role in protecting against cataract formation.[169] The study of 1380 people who attended an ophthalmology outpatient clinic which I mentioned on page 111 found that regular use of multivitamin supplements, including riboflavin, decreased the risk of developing cataracts by 37 per cent.[170]

Where you find it

Dietary sources include yeast extract, liver, wholegrain cereals, dairy products, eggs, green leafy vegetables and beans. Riboflavin is easily lost from food. Two hours' exposure to sunlight destroys the riboflavin content of a bottle of milk by 90 per cent, for example, so buy milk in cartons rather than bottles.

How much you need

The new EU RDA is 1.4mg. People who are physically active need more riboflavin than those who take little regular exercise; a nutritional therapist may suggest 25 to 100mg. Older people and those with diabetes need to obtain more B2 from their diet to maintain blood levels.

As excess B2 is excreted in the urine, the colour of your urine may become noticeably more yellow when you take supplements containing riboflavin.

Side effects/safety

There are no serious concerns about taking B2 at recommended doses.

Vitamin B3 (niacin)

What it is

Vitamin B3 is a water-soluble vitamin that exists in two forms: nicotinic acid and nicotinamide. Small amounts of B3 can be made in the body from the essential amino acid tryptophan, but not enough to meet our daily needs.

How it can help you

Vitamin B3 works together with the mineral chromium (see page 176) to form the organic complex 'glucose tolerance factor'. GTF, and therefore vitamin B3, is essential for the action of insulin in controlling glucose uptake by cells, and also plays an important role in releasing glycogen from your muscles for use as energy and for processing fatty acids released from body fat stores. It works together with vitamins B1 and B2 to increase energy production in cells.

Lowering cholesterol levels Vitamin B3 is prescribed to help lower abnormally high cholesterol levels. At high doses (under medical supervision) it has been shown to reduce the risk of both non-fatal and fatal heart attacks by as much as 30 per cent. Niacin is now recognised as the most effective treatment available to increase levels of beneficial HDL cholesterol.[171] It can also lower total cholesterol, harmful LDL cholesterol and triglycerides as well as being one of the few treatments that can lower a harmful type of fat particle known as apolipoprotein (apo) B, and of another fat, apoA.[172] It seems to work in the liver to reduce production of triglycerides and apoB, while also blocking the reactions that break down HDL cholesterol.

In one 16-week trial involving 148 people with diabetes, a once-daily slow-release B3 supplement was shown to increase beneficial HDL cholesterol levels by 19 to 24 per cent compared with a placebo, and to lower triglyceride levels by 13 to 28 per cent. And it achieved this with no significant changes to glucose control or HbA1c levels.[173]

Where you find it

You can find niacin in wheat and maize flour, meat, eggs, milk and yeast extract.

In the UK, flour is fortified with vitamin B3 to replace the amounts lost through processing.

How much you need

The new EU RDA is 16mg, but people who are physically active need more niacin. Higher doses of 50mg or more per day may be prescribed for certain medical disorders such as raised cholesterol levels (see above). Regular blood tests are then usually needed to check liver function.

Supplements may describe their vitamin B3 content as 'niacin equivalents'. These are equal to the amount of nicotinamide and nicotinic acid they contain, plus one-sixtieth of the amount of tryptophan (an amino acid) they contain – as some can be converted into B3 in the body.

Side effects/safety

High-dose niacin (above 30mg, and especially in the form of nicotinic acid) can cause facial blushing because of the vitamin's ability to dilate the veins. If you're out and about and want to take a niacin supplement, a low dose of aspirin (75 to 300mg) taken half an hour before you have your B3 can reduce the blushing effect.

Very high doses of niacin can cause symptoms of toxicity – which may include the worsening of conditions such as diabetes, as well as thickening and darkening of patches of skin, palpitations, peptic ulcers, gout and hepatitis.

Niacin may affect folic acid metabolism, and increase levels of homocysteine in the blood[174] (see page 152). It may therefore be sensible to take niacin in combination with B6, B12 and folic acid.

Trials have shown that people with diabetes can safely use niacin, as it does not have adverse effects on glucose control. It may even produce a significant fall in HbA1c levels.[175] Niacin can also be used together with a statin drug, which lowers LDL cholesterol in a different way.

Vitamin B6 (pyridoxine)

What it is

Natural vitamin B6 is actually a group of water-soluble substances, including pyridoxine, pyridoxal and pyridoxamine, which are all converted to the most active form, pyridoxine, in the body.

How it can help you

Pyridoxine is essential for the proper functioning of over 60 enzymes in the body. You need it to synthesise genetic material, amino acids and proteins, and to metabolise body stores of carbo-hydrate (glycogen) and essential fatty acids.

Regular supplies of vitamin B6 are needed by rapidly dividing cells such as those found in the gut, skin, hair follicles and marrow. It is sometimes called the immune booster, as it's key to the cells that produce antibodies and fight infection, known as lympho-cytes. One of B6's most important roles is its involvement in the breakdown of homocysteine, which at high levels, as you'll remember, can damage artery walls and increase the risk of coronary heart disease (see page 152).

Preventing coronary heart disease In the Nurses' Health Study,[176] which I have mentioned in other contexts, a total of 80,082 women with no previous history of coronary heart disease, cancer, high cholesterol levels or diabetes completed a detailed food questionnaire. Their intake of nutrients was then assessed. Over 14 years of follow-up, the number of heart attacks were recorded as well as factors such as smoking, high blood pressure, and the amount of alcohol, fat and fibre they consumed.

Those with the highest intakes of vitamin B6 were 45 per cent less likely to have a heart attack than those with the lowest. The researchers concluded that an intake of vitamin B6 above the current recommended dietary allowance may be important in the prevention of coronary heart disease in women. The most likely mechanism is the vitamin's ability to lower homocysteine levels in the blood.

Lowering risk for peripheral vascular disease Developing peripheral vascular disease (page 33) is a risk for people with diabetes. In one study involving 392 men over the age of 50, of whom 22 per cent had the disease,[177] the researchers found that intakes of vitamin B6 were lower in these men, along with their levels of folate consumption. The researchers concluded that low levels of folate and vitamin B6 were independent risk factors for peripheral vascular disease after taking other risk factors such as age, blood pressure, cholesterol levels, diabetes, and smoking status into account.

Alleviating diabetic neuropathy Lack of vitamin B6 has been linked with nerve damage, although this finding remains controversial. In one study, vitamin B6 levels were measured in 50 people who had diabetic neuropathy (see page 27) and found to be significantly lower than in a group of people with diabetes who did not have neuropathy.[178]

A deficiency in vitamin B6 has also been linked with carpal tunnel syndrome, in which tendons in the wrist become inflamed. However, when B6 levels were measured in 13 people with both diabetes and carpal tunnel syndrome, no significant differences were found between those with carpal tunnel syndrome, diabetics without neuropathy, and healthy people.[179] This suggests that carpal tunnel syndrome in people with diabetes may not be the result of low levels of B6.

Alleviating diabetic retinopathy Vitamin B6 may help to reduce retinopathy (see page 24) in people with diabetes. This observation is backed by a study following 18 people with diabetes for up to 28 years. Those who took vitamin B6 supplements did not develop retinopathy. The researchers described this discovery as 'monumental' and in need of further investigation.[180]

Where you find it

Food sources of vitamin B6 include wholegrains, liver meat, oily fish, soy products, bananas, nuts (especially walnuts), green leafy vegetables, avocados and egg yolk. Yeast extract and royal jelly are also good sources. Vitamin B6 is easily destroyed by cooking and exposure to light.

How much you need

The new EU RDA for vitamin B6 is 2mg. Higher doses of 10 to 200mg may be suggested by nutritional therapists, as some studies have found that people with type 2 diabetes tend to have lower levels of vitamin B6 compared with non-diabetics.[181] In two studies, blood levels of vitamin B6 were found to be low in 25 per cent of 518 adults with type 2 diabetes and 24 per cent of 63 children with type 1 diabetes.[182,183]

Side effects/safety

The risks associated with taking B6 at doses between 10 and 200mg long term are unclear, but are probably low; although some think it may cause nerve symptoms such as pins and needles, this is not definitely proven. Taking vitamin 40mg twice daily for three weeks does not appear to affect glucose control in people with diabetes, as no changes have been found in either oral glucose tolerance tests or insulin response to glucose.[184]

In another study, taking 50mg of B6 three times daily for six weeks was also found to have no effect on blood glucose levels, but did reduce the level of glycosylated HbA1c by around 6 per cent.[185] This suggests that vitamin B6 may reduce glycosylation of proteins (see page 22). If this is correct, this may be another role in which it helps to reduce complications of diabetes in addition to its role lowering homocysteine levels.

Vitamin B12 (cyanocobalamin)

What it is

Vitamin B12 is a water-soluble vitamin which can be stored in the liver. This means we usually have enough to last several years. The vitamin is absorbed in the lower part of the small intestine, but only if a carrier protein, 'intrinsic factor', is present. B12 deficiency sometimes develops in later life because of a lack of intrinsic factor or disease of the small intestine.

Ten to 30 per cent of people with type 2 diabetes who are taking metformin for glucose control showed evidence of reduced vitamin B12 absorption but, as absorption of vitamin B12 is dependent on calcium, taking calcium supplements has been shown to reverse this metformin-induced fall in vitamin B12 absorption.[186]

B12 is essential for the synthesis of DNA during cell division. When B12 is in short supply, dividing cells become unusually large; and if this happens to red blood cells, pernicious anaemia – the symptoms of which tend to creep up over a long time – can result. This has relevance for people with type 1 diabetes, as one study showed the prevalence of pernicious anaemia in people with both type 1 diabetes and autoimmune thyroid disease to be as high as 6.3 per cent in one study, with females being slightly more at risk.[187]

Vitamin B12 is also needed for healthy nerve function, and an uncorrected deficiency can lead to spinal cord damage, although this is rare.

How it can help you

Together with folic acid and vitamin B6, B12 is important for lowering homocysteine levels (see page 155), and also plays a role in protecting against some congenital abnormalities, such as spina bifida.

Alleviating diabetic retinopathy Raised levels of homocysteine have been linked with an increased risk of proliferative retinopathy – the advanced form of diabetic retinopathy (see page 25) – in people with type 2 diabetes.[188] This condition might be expected to improve with the addition of B12, folic acid and B6, due to their beneficial effects on homocysteine levels.

Interestingly, treating diabetic retinopathy with vitamin B12 was tried as far back as the 1950s – before homocysteine was even known about – but these studies do not seem to have received much follow-up. In one early study, 100mcg B12 was added to insulin injections given to 15 people with retinopathy as a complication of type 1 diabetes.[189] A year later, the retinopathy was said to have disappeared in seven of the participants. Similar results were also reported in another study from the same year.[190]

Where you find it

Food sources of vitamin B12 include liver, kidney, meat, oily fish (especially sardines), eggs and dairy products. Supplements supplying synthetic B12, or natural forms derived from blue-green algae or bacterial cultures, are available for vegetarians.

How much you need

The new EU RDA for B12 is 2.5mcg. Intakes as high as 2mg per day appear to be safe. Although vitamin B12 as a treatment for pernicious anaemia is traditionally given as regular injections, it can also be given orally in a very high dose (up to 2mg a day).

Side effects/safety

No serious side effects have been reported as any excess is excreted in the urine. As vitamin B12 deficiency can be masked by taking folate supplements, these two vitamins are usually given together.

Folic acid

What it is

Folic acid is a water-soluble vitamin. It is the synthetic form of the naturally occurring folate, and is actually preferable in supplements as it is more readily absorbed and used more efficiently in the body.

How it can help you

Folic acid is involved in the synthesis and metabolism of proteins, sugar and nucleic acids during cell division. Like vitamin B12, it is needed in particular by cells that are in the process of dividing rapidly. When folic acid is in short supply, newly formed chromosomes are more likely to be abnormal and cells – especially red blood cells – become larger than normal which can, as we have seen, lead to pernicious anaemia.

Folic acid is also essential during the first few weeks of a baby's development in the womb, to help prevent a type of developmental abnormality known as a neural tube defect (such as spina bifida) which arises between the 24th and 28th day after conception. Because of its effects on cell division, folic acid may also help to protect against certain cancers, including cancers of the cervix, oesophagus, mouth (especially in smokers), colon and rectum, as well as smoking-related cancers of the lung, and breast cancer in women with a high alcohol intake.

Two of the three enzymes that control homocysteine levels depend on folic acid for their activity – so this vitamin can also cut the risk of stroke and coronary heart disease.

Reducing coronary heart disease In the 14 years of follow-up to the Nurses' Health Study,[191] the number of heart attacks in the over 80,000 women participating were recorded, along with factors such as smoking, high blood pressure, and intakes of alcohol, fat and fibre. It was found that those with the highest intakes of folate were 45 per cent less likely to have a heart attack than those with the lowest. The conclusion was that taking folate above the current recommended dietary allowance may be important in the prevention of coronary heart disease in women.

In another study of a group of 82 people with diabetes, those who had existing cardiovascular disease had levels of homocysteine significantly higher than those without cardiovascular disease.[192] They were also more likely to have low levels of folic acid. In this particular study of people with diabetes, the level of homocysteine was found to be dependent on the level of folic acid rather than vitamin B12.

Lowering risk of peripheral vascular disease As was shown in the study (see page 164) of 392 men over 50 years old, including 86 with peripheral vascular disease (see page 33),[193] daily intakes of folate and vitamin B6 are independent risk factors for the disease, after taking other factors such as age, blood pressure, cholesterol levels, diabetes and smoking status into account.

Intermittent claudication – a pain in the calves that comes on during exercise as a result of peripheral vascular disease – is relatively common in older people with diabetes. In one study of over 15,000 middle-aged men without diabetes, researchers found that levels of homocysteine were significantly higher in those with intermittent claudication than in those without.[194] High homocysteine levels were also found to occur mainly in those with low folic acid levels. This suggests that people with intermittent claudication should take folic acid supplements.

Lowering blood pressure A study involving 33 people with type 2 diabetes and 16 healthy volunteers found links between folic acid levels, homocysteine and systolic arterial blood pressure (the highest pressure in the arteries as the heart beats).[195] Patients with raised homocysteine levels had significantly higher diastolic blood pressure (the lowest pressure in the arteries, as the heart rests between beats). Those without raised homocysteine levels had higher folic acid levels, which were in their turn associated with lower systolic blood pressure. It is highly likely that the raised homocysteine levels associated with low folic acid levels damage artery linings and affect their flexibility, leading to raised blood pressure.[196]

Preventing stroke In one study, almost 44,000 men aged 40 to 75 years who were initially free of cardiovascular diseases and diabetes were followed for 14 years, from 1986 to 2000.[197] Their diets were assessed every four years, and after adjustment for other lifestyle and dietary factors, it was found that those with the highest intake of folic acid had a significantly lower risk of ischemic stroke, which results when a brain artery becomes blocked, although not haemorrhagic stroke, which is triggered by a ruptured blood vessel. B12 was also important in reducing risk of ischemic stroke.

Preventing cataracts A study found that people with the highest intake of folic acid are 60 per cent less likely to develop cataracts severe enough to need surgery, compared to those with the lowest intakes.[198]

Where you find it

Folate (the natural form of folic acid) is found in green leafy vegetables such as spinach, broccoli and Brussels sprouts, and in wholegrains, beans, soya products, liver, kidney, some fruits and nuts and dairy products. It is difficult to obtain optimum amounts of folate from dietary sources alone, however: foods originally rich in folate may have less than a third of it left after processing and cooking. So supplementation with folic acid is probably a wise move.

How much you need

The RDA for folic acid is 200mcg. Women planning a baby should take 400mcg folic acid a day (or 4mg, if they have a personal or family history of conceiving a child with a neural tube defect such as spina bifida).

High levels of homocysteine (see page 152) can also be reduced by taking folic acid supplements. People with a family or personal history of coronary heart disease may be advised to take at least 400mcg folic acid daily.

Your body stores very little folic acid and dietary lack rapidly causes deficiency – it is probably the most widespread vitamin deficiency in developed countries. Some studies have found that people with type 2 diabetes tend to have lower levels of folic acid compared to people without diabetes.[199] Drinking excess alcohol may also lower your levels of folic acid.

Side effects/safety

Taking some anti-epilepsy drugs can lower levels of folic acid. People taking drugs to treat epilepsy should tell their doctor if they take folic acid supplements so blood levels of their medication can be monitored where appropriate. For women on anti-epileptic drugs who want to have a baby, it is vitally important to contact their doctor about taking extra folic acid supplements. Folic acid should usually be taken together with vitamin B12. This is because lack of vitamin B12 (which leads to damage of the nervous system, especially the spinal cord) is masked by taking folic acid supplements (as this prevents the occurrence of pernicious anaemia, which usually allows lack of vitamin B12 to be detected).

Folic acid is generally considered safe, even at doses as high as 1 to 5mg per day. However, as it may mask vitamin B12 deficiency, the usual recommended upper dose of folic acid is normally set at 1mg daily. For those with high levels of homocysteine or a high risk of conceiving a child with a neural tube defect, doses of 5mg per day or more may be advised – if you've been tested and this sounds like you, seek medical advice and take doses like this only under medical supervision.

Biotin

What it is

Biotin is a water-soluble B group vitamin needed for the synthesis and metabolism of glucose, fatty acids, amino acids, genetic material and stress hormones.

How it can help you

Improving glucose control Biotin can improve glucose metabolism by stimulating the secretion of insulin from beta cells and increasing the breakdown of glucose in the liver and pancreas. Researchers therefore suspect it may improve the metabolism and use of glucose in people with type 2 diabetes,[200] although to date there does not seem to be a lot of published human research in this area – somewhat surprisingly.

One study looked at whether large doses of biotin, given intravenously to people undergoing dialysis, could improve their oral glucose tolerance test. This study was undertaken because people with renal failure often have an abnormal glucose metabolism linked with insulin resistance, putting them at risk of diabetes type 2. Eleven people without diabetes, who were undergoing dialysis three times a week, had their fasting blood glucose and glycosylated haemoglobin measured before and two hours after receiving 75g of glucose (by drinking a sugary solution as part of an oral glucose tolerance test – see page 15). These measurements were made before, two weeks after and two months after receiving 50mg of biotin by injection directly into a vein.[201] The glucose tolerance test was abnormal in four people before they received the biotin injections, but three of these people became normal afterwards – indicating that biotin may be beneficial for glucose control in people at risk of developing type 2 diabetes.

In another study, seven people with type 1 diabetes stopped taking insulin for one week, during which they were given either high-dose biotin (16mg per day) or a placebo. In those on the placebo, fasting blood glucose levels rose; but in those receiving biotin, blood glucose levels decreased significantly.[202] Yet another study showed that biotin levels in the blood were significantly lower in 43 patients with type 2 diabetes than in healthy controls, and that lower fasting blood glucose levels were associated with higher blood biotin levels. When 9mg of biotin per day was supplemented, their fasting blood glucose levels fell by an average of 45 per cent[203] but did not change in those receiving the placebo.

Treating peripheral neuropathy Three people with severe diabetic peripheral neuropathy – affecting nerves other than those in the brain and spinal cord – were given 10mg of biotin daily by injection for six weeks, then 10mg by injection three times a week for six weeks, then 5mg per day by mouth for one to three years.[204] Within four to eight weeks of treatment, they reported significant improvements in symptoms which were confirmed by clinical and laboratory findings. The researchers suggest that diabetes may be associated with a deficiency, inactivity or unavailability of biotin, resulting in the abnormal metabolism of carbo-

172

hydrates within nerve cells. They went as far as to suggest that regular biotin administration should be recommended for every diabetic person to help prevent and treat peripheral neuropathy, although extensive randomised clinical trials are needed first.

Where you find it

Food sources include meat, liver, oily fish, egg yolk, wholegrains, nuts, some vegetables such as cauliflower plus yeast extract. As biotin is widely distributed in food, and is also made by bacteria in the gut, from which it can be absorbed, a serious dietary deficiency is rare. Taking long-term antibiotics can deplete biotin, however, so it's a good idea to invest in probiotics (see page 117) if you have to take a course of antibiotics. Biotin deficiency can also occur in people, such as bodybuilders, who eat large amounts of raw egg white over a long period. Raw, but not cooked, egg white contains a protein called avidin that binds to biotin in the gut and prevents its absorption.

How much you need

The new EU RDA for biotin is 0.05mg (equivalent to 50mcg). If you have neuropathy, or want help with your glucose control, taking up to 1mg daily may be recommended. No serious side effects have been reported.

One in every 123 people is estimated to have an inherited condition related to biotin metabolism – either a deficiency of the enzyme biotinidase, or impaired action in another enzyme, holocarboxylase. This is believed to affect their immunity against yeast infections. If this is the case, taking high-dose biotin supplements will solve the problem.[205]

Minerals

It's strange to think that we carry around 3 whole kilograms of minerals and trace elements in our bodies, most of it in our bones and teeth. But minerals don't just shore up our internal scaffolding. Like vitamins, they are dynamic players within the body, and about 20 minerals and trace elements – those needed in tiny amounts only – are essential for the biochemical reactions that take place during metabolism. Even more to the point, a number of minerals are emerging as key for controlling aspects of diabetes such as glucose tolerance, as well as serious associated conditions – high levels of blood fats and coronary heart disease, for instance.

Here are some of the roles minerals play in your body:

- calcium, magnesium and phosphate keep your internal framework – bones and teeth – in sound working order
- sodium, potassium and calcium maintain normal cell function
- copper, iron, magnesium, manganese, molybdenum, selenium and zinc act as co-factors for important enzymes, helping them function properly
- iron aids oxygen transport
- chromium and iodine regulate hormone function
- selenium and manganese act as antioxidants.

Some trace elements such as nickel, tin and vanadium are known to be essential for normal growth, although their exact roles are not yet fully understood.

A number of minerals are beneficial for people with diabetes, especially:

- Chromium – which plays an important role in regulating blood glucose levels in people with type 2 diabetes, as it interacts with insulin to help glucose enter muscle and fat cells. It may only help people who are chromium deficient but, as this is relatively common, there is little harm in trying a chromium supplement at a dose of at least 200mcg daily for a few months to see if it helps.
- Copper – choose a multivitamin and mineral supplement which includes copper as many people are copper deficient, and it does seem to help glucose control in people with type 2 diabetes.
- Magnesium – which affects how well insulin works to control glucose levels; it has even been suggested that magnesium deficiency may contribute to the development of metabolic syndrome, type 2 diabetes and some diabetic complications such as foot ulceration. Magnesium is also beneficial for the heart and circulation.
- Zinc – which has been shown to improve insulin production and its effectiveness and may help to reduce the risk of some complications such as foot ulceration.

In this chapter we'll be looking only at the minerals that are proving to have a major impact on diabetes and health problems associated with it. (Selenium, which also has major antioxidant action, is covered in Chapter 8.)

You'll need to know about them because you can only obtain minerals and trace elements from your diet. As a result, mineral deficiencies are more common than vitamin deficiencies, especially if you eat vegetables grown in mineral-poor soils. Acid rain and food processing can also reduce the mineral content of foods.

Minerals are best taken as part of a multivitamin and mineral formulation rather than by taking them individually, although some people with diabetes may be advised to take a chromium or magnesium supplement in higher dose than that found in a standard A-Z type formula.

Now let's look at each of these vital substances in detail.

Chromium

··

What it is

Chromium is important in several ways. It regulates your metabolism and helps synthesise fatty acids; but most vitally for you, as a diabetic, it helps balance insulin and blood sugar. Along with niacin and certain amino acids, chromium goes to form an organic complex known as the glucose tolerance factor or GTF, which interacts with insulin to help carry glucose out of your bloodstream and into your cells.

Interestingly, your chromium levels rapidly decrease after birth, especially after the age of 10. Your levels then fall as you get older.[206] Some experts believe this finding reflects a widespread nutritional deficiency in this important trace element, which may be related to premature ageing.[207]

How it can help you

A lot of evidence points to the vital importance of chromium in combating or treating diabetes. It's significant, for instance, that lower chromium levels have been found in people with diabetes,[208] and also that their level of chromium in white blood cells is much lower than in their blood plasma.[209] This dearth of chromium in cells reflects a general deficiency, whereas the higher amounts in the plasma could mean that chromium is lost through the kidneys to contribute to that overall deficiency. One study found that people with type 2 diabetes lose as much as double the amount of chromium in their urine as healthy people do.[210]

Glucose tolerance factor, or GTF, doesn't just aid the uptake of glucose by cells. It also encourages the production of energy from glucose, especially in muscles; increases protein synthesis; and lowers blood fat levels, including those of harmful LDL cholesterol. It may also suppress hunger pangs by directly affecting the part of the brain that registers satiety. Chromium appears to have a useful antioxidant action in people with type 2 diabetes, too.[211]

Encouraging glucose tolerance Low levels of chromium have been linked with poor glucose tolerance[212,213,214,215] and diabetes, and it is now widely believed that a lack of chromium in the diet is a risk factor for type 2 diabetes in some people. Although this was suspected back in the 1960s, the first confirmation came in 1977, when a patient on long-term intravenous feeding who developed severe diabetes and neuropathy was cured after chromium was added to her intravenous food.[216]

It is now known that chromium has a beneficial effect on the interactions between glucose, insulin and glucagon – a hormone that raises the level of blood glucose – to improve glucose tolerance. Chromium acts on certain receptor sites on cells – the spots where insulin binds to them before it escorts the glucose in – and so increases insulin sensitivity in the body.[217] Some researchers have suggested that the increase in chromium deficiency seen with age may be an important underlying cause of type 2 diabetes in some people, although this is controversial.[218]

In one interesting study,[219] 180 people with type 2 diabetes were given either 100mcg chromium picolinate (a patented, widely sold form that combines chromium with picolinic acid), 500mcg chromium picolinate or a placebo twice a day. After two and four months, those receiving a total of 1000mcg chromium daily showed consistent improvements in fasting glucose, fasting insulin, improvements in glucose and insulin levels after a meal, and their glycosylated HbA1c, indicating better long-term glucose control. Glucose control didn't improve in those taking 200mcg a day, but reductions in insulin levels when these people were fasting and after eating were as good as those achieved on 1000mcg a day.

Some people with type 1 diabetes may also benefit from chromium if they are receiving insulin injections but have a degree of insulin resistance. There is one report[220] of a woman who at 28 had had type 1 diabetes for 18 years, and whose need for insulin was increasing. When given 200mcg chromium picolinate twice daily for three months, her glucose level and glycosylated haemoglobin concentrations improved.

In another study, when supplements providing 200mcg chromium per day were given to people with diabetes, nearly half needed less insulin or blood sugar-lowering tablets. The people with non-insulin dependent diabetes responded much better than those with insulin-dependent diabetes.

Some trials have found little improvement in glucose tolerance through chromium supplementation, however.[221] It may only be of benefit where there is both insulin resistance and a deficiency of chromium in the diet. It should be noted that trials showing poor results for chromium in this context have tended to use chromium chloride, which has such poor absorption and bioavailability that it is now rarely used. It's also possible that volunteers had low niacin levels, which you may remember is a component of GTF – and therefore a crucial player in chromium's efficacy in the body.

The findings on chromium and glucose tolerance do remain inconclusive and further studies are undoubtedly needed. But given the safety of taking sensible amounts of chromium, its use is widely recommended for people with diabetes, for its potentially beneficial effects.

Lowering blood fat levels It's been found that chromium levels in people with coronary heart disease are lower than in healthy people, and chromium deficiency may be an independent risk factor for cardiovascular disease.[222] So chromium supplements may help to reduce the risk of coronary heart disease by lowering blood levels of harmful triglycerides and raising levels of beneficial HDL cholesterol.

In one study[223] involving 78 people with type 2 diabetes, half were given brewer's yeast, which contains chromium, followed by 200mcg of chromium chloride, with a placebo in between, for four eight-week stages. Both supplements reduced triglyceride levels, while average beneficial HDL cholesterol levels increased. In some cases, people previously needing insulin injections no longer required them. The researchers concluded that chromium supplements produced better blood fat control (along with better glucose control), and lowered the need for drug treatment in people with type 2 diabetes. Similar beneficial effects on triglyceride and HDL cholesterol levels from taking chromium chloride were found in another study involving 76 people with established arterial disease, some of whom had type 2.[224]

In another study,[225] 30 people with type 2 diabetes took either 200mcg chromium picolinate or a placebo every day for two months. Then, after a two-month period with nothing, the researchers reversed whatever they had been taking. It was found that while on chromium picolinate, the participants' triglyceride levels fell significantly by 17.4 per cent. The team concluded that the low cost and excellent safety profile of chromium make it an attractive option for lowering levels of blood fats.

Encouraging weight loss Because chromium affects appetite, hunger pangs and fat metabolism, it is used in some weight-loss products – and could be of interest to you if you have metabolic syndrome or type 2 diabetes and are eager to shed some pounds.

In one study,[226] 233 people received either 200 or 400mcg of chromium or a placebo a day for 72 days. They were given no dietary or exercise advice and could follow whichever type of weight-loss programme they wanted to.

At the beginning of the trial, there were no significant differences in weight, or in the amounts of body fat and lean mass, between the three groups. After the trial, body composition improvements, or BCI, were calculated based on losses in body fat and increases in lean body mass (mainly muscle). Those receiving the placebo only lost 0.4kg, while those on the chromium lost an average of 1.26kg. And, when their BCI was calculated, those taking the chromium lost more fat compared with lean body mass. These differences are highly significant.

So, when combined with a sensible diet and regular exercise, chromium supplements may help some people to lose weight, especially if they have insulin resistance and are deficient in chromium. Other studies have shown little benefit, however, and it is evident that more research is needed.

Where you find it

Foods containing chromium include egg yolk, red meat, cheese, fruit and fruit juice, wholegrains, honey, vegetables and condiments such as black pepper and thyme. As plants do not need chromium, the chromium content of fruit and vegetables depends entirely on the amount and type of the mineral in the soil where the plants are grown.

Processing can reduce the mineral content of foods by up to 80 per cent. Most refined grains, for instance, have little chromium content. Brewer's yeast is a particularly good source of chromium as it is already in the form of GTF, making it at least 10 times more effective than that obtained from other food sources. Special chromium-enriched yeast strains have now been developed.

How much you need

The new EU RDA for chromium is 40mcg with intakes of up to 10mg from both diet and supplements thought to produce no harmful ill effects. On average, however, those following a Westernised diet obtain much less than this. One study of 22 'well-balanced' diets found that the chromium level in it was, on average, just 13.4mcg per day.[227]

In fact, chromium deficiency is thought to be common. One estimate suggested that 90 per cent of adults are deficient, as most people get less than 50mcg from their diet, and only around 2 per cent of this is in an absorbable form.

In general, the more carbohydrate you eat, the more chromium you need. Chromium supplements are best absorbed when taken with vitamin C, while supplements containing calcium will reduce absorption.

Inorganic chromium is best combined with vitamin B3 (niacin) to ensure that it is incorporated into GTF.[228] So taking chromium nicotinate supplements, rather than chromium chloride, will do the job for you.

Side effects/safety

Chromium appears to be the safest of nutritional minerals. Although there has been a scare based on findings in fruit flies, chromium chloride and chromium picolinate have been given to rats at doses that are thousands of times higher than those used weight-for-weight in humans, with no evidence of toxicity.[229] The US Institute of Medicine did not find any credible basis for setting an upper dose limit for chromium picolinate, although the European authorities took a more cautious view by excluding it from the EU Directive on Food Supplements. The UK Food Standards Agency have suggested introducing a ban, which seems ludicrous based on the current evidence.

It's important, however, not to exceed the above recommended dose for chromium, as otherwise it may interfere with zinc and iron absorption.

Copper

What it is

Copper is a trace element needed to produce a number of brain chemicals, the skin pigment melanin and the red blood pigment haemoglobin. It plays an important role in oxygen transportation; is essential for the function of a number of antioxidant enzymes; and is needed for the metabolism of vitamin C. This means, however, that if vitamin C intakes are good, a copper deficiency can quickly occur. One study of 83 people with type 2 diabetes found that copper levels were significantly higher compared with those of non-diabetics.[230]

How it can help you

Encouraging glucose tolerance In animal studies, copper deficiency is associated with impaired glucose tolerance[231] and elevated levels of glycosylated HbA1c.[232] One study[233] found a significant difference in copper levels in women with type 1 diabetes compared with healthy volunteers, whether or not they had good glucose control. For men, however, the only significant differences found were between the healthy subjects and men with type 1 and poor glucose control. They did not find a significant link between copper levels and HbA1c.

In another study, two men who had a low intake of just 0.7 to 0.8mg copper per day for five to six months developed higher glucose levels. Their levels returned to normal after the researchers boosted their intake of copper.[234] In a similar trial[235] involving two other volunteers, a dose of 6mg copper per day improved their response to an oral glucose tolerance test, suggesting that their usual diet was copper-deficient.

Preventing coronary heart disease A lack of copper has been suggested as a cause of coronary heart disease,[236] initially in 1973.[237] Since that time, copper deficiency has been shown to impair glucose tolerance; promote abnormal blood clotting; increase blood pressure; and adversely affect heart rhythms.[238] Interestingly, dietary copper is around a hundred times more effective in lowering cholesterol levels than the cholesterol-lowering drug, clofibrate.[239] It has therefore been suggested that dietary copper intake may be a powerful determinant of raised cholesterol.

Copper's effect on the heart and on phenomena associated with heart health, such as cholesterol, doesn't stop there. An enzyme called copper-zinc superoxide dismutase is dependent on copper for its activity, and provides important antioxidant protection against free radicals. It has therefore been suggested that copper is an antioxidant nutrient for heart and circulatory health.[240] Low levels of copper have also been found to raise homocysteine levels, while high homocysteine levels interfere with the body's ability to make use of copper. Not everyone agrees with the research linking adequate copper to a healthy heart, however. Some researchers suggest excess copper is a leading cause of atherosclerosis – especially where the person is not getting enough antioxidants. This possibility was investigated in 4574 people, of whom 151 later died from coronary heart disease.[241] At the start of the study, copper levels were found to be 5 per cent higher among those who died from coronary heart disease. After taking other factors such as age, sex, smoking status, blood pressure, cholesterol levels, HDL cholesterol, weight, exercise and history of diabetes into account, those with the highest copper levels were found to be 2.87 times more likely to have a heart attack than those with the lower levels.

Another study[242] suggested that high copper levels are an independent risk factor for coronary heart disease. Copper levels were assessed in 1666 randomly selected males who did not have coronary heart disease at the start of the trial. It was found that those with the highest copper levels were 3.5 to 4 times more likely to go on to have a heart attack than those with the lowest levels.

It's a confusing picture, and further research is undoubtedly needed to unravel whether a deficiency or excess of copper increases the risk of coronary heart disease.

Where you find it

Dietary sources of copper include crustaceans such as prawns, shellfish (especially oysters), olives, nuts, pulses and wholegrains. It is also present in green vegetables grown in copper-rich soil. Up to 70 per cent of our dietary intake remains unabsorbed, however, as it stays bound to other bowel contents.

How much you need

The new EU RDA for copper is 1mg with intakes of up to 10mg from both diet and supplements thought to produce no harmful ill effects. One leading authority[243] believes that the lack of a recommended daily intake is harmful to health. Men and women fed diets containing only around 1mg copper a day (which is fairly typical for a Western diet) develop reversible, but potentially harmful changes in blood pressure control, cholesterol and glucose metabolism, as well as showing changes in heart rhythm. As we saw above, such a deficiency may – although arguably – lead to coronary heart disease.

Many of the adverse effects of excess zinc (see page 194) are due to interference with copper metabolism leading to a relative copper deficiency. The ideal dietary ratio of copper to zinc is 1:10 – commonly found in supplements. It's worth checking labels to ensure the ratio is not widely different from this.

Side effects/safety

If you take just twice the recommended amount of copper, or if your water is supplied through copper pipes, you can be at risk of developing an excess of this mineral. This can be toxic, causing restlessness, nausea, vomiting, colic and diarrhoea. Taking too much copper over the long term can lead to copper-induced cirrhosis of the liver.

Magnesium
....

What it is

Our bones and teeth hold some 70 per cent of the essential mineral magnesium. Magnesium is also important for maintaining the electrical stability of cells, and is vital for controlling the entry of calcium into heart cells, which ensures a regular heartbeat. But it doesn't stop there. Magnesium is an essential player in every major metabolic reaction, from the synthesis of protein and genetic material to the production of energy from glucose. Few enzymes can work without it.

How it can help you

If you are overweight, obese or have metabolic syndrome, there is some very heartening new research suggesting that a diet rich in magnesium may actually help to prevent the development of type 2 diabetes. Researchers in the US analysed the dietary health of 85,060 women and 42,872 men with no history of diabetes.[244] After following them for 12 to 18 years, they found that those with the largest dietary intake of magnesium were least likely to develop diabetes. Another study[245] looked at 39,345 women, and found that in those who were overweight, the ones who consumed the highest amounts of magnesium were 22 per cent less likely to develop type 2 diabetes than those with the lowest intakes.

Improving glucose tolerance People with diabetes tend to have low levels of magnesium, and this essential mineral is intimately linked with the workings of insulin. It has, in fact, been found that people taking adequate amounts of magnesium – usually from supplements – are less likely to develop type 2 diabetes.

Magnesium concentrations in the body are usually tightly controlled by several factors, including insulin levels; these affect how much magnesium is found inside each cell. In its turn, the level of magnesium inside a cell has been shown to affect how well insulin controls glucose levels, and insulin requirements appear to be lower in people with type 1 diabetes who take magnesium supplements.[246] The low magnesium levels found in diabetes may worsen insulin resistance in people with type 2 diabetes and/or high blood pressure. It has even been suggested that low levels of magnesium in cells could be the missing link between type 2 diabetes and high blood pressure.[247]

In one large trial,[248] the magnesium intake and levels of over 12,000 non-diabetic people were assessed, and studied for six years. The white – but not the black – people with the lowest magnesium levels were found to be twice as likely to develop type 2 diabetes over this time. Recently, magnesium levels in 192 people with metabolic syndrome were also assessed and compared with those in 384 similar people without metabolic syndrome. Low magnesium levels were found in 65.6 per cent of those with metabolic syndrome, compared with only 4.9 per cent of those without. Those with low magnesium levels were 6.8 times more likely to have metabolic syndrome, 2.8 times more likely to have abnormal blood fat levels and almost twice as likely to have high blood pressure.[249]

In another trial, 63 people with type 2 diabetes and low magnesium levels took either 2.6g magnesium chloride supplements or a placebo daily for 16 weeks. Those receiving magnesium supplements showed significant improvements in glucose levels, insulin sensitivity and HbA1c levels compared with those on the placebo.[250]

Preventing coronary heart disease A study involving over 15,000 people found that magnesium levels were significantly lower in people with coronary heart disease, high blood pressure and diabetes. Low magnesium levels were also linked to high fasting insulin and glucose levels, and low dietary intakes of magnesium were associated with high insulin and LDL cholesterol levels and, in women, with thickened walls in the carotid artery, which supplies blood to the head.[251]

It's known, in fact, that a lack of magnesium causes the coronary arteries to progressively constrict, reducing the amount of oxygen and nutrients reaching heart muscle cells. So it has been found that correcting levels of magnesium has a beneficial effect on the heart and circulation.[252]

As for cholesterol, one study[253] suggested that magnesium supplementation can help in treating raised cholesterol levels in people with type 2 diabetes. Twenty-six people with type 2 diabetes were given magnesium supplements for a month, and 17 people received a placebo. The people who took the magnesium supplements significantly reduced their total cholesterol and LDL cholesterol, and boosted levels of beneficial HDL cholesterol.

Reducing risk of diabetic foot ulcers Low magnesium levels increase the risk of neuropathy (see page 27) and abnormal blood clotting, both of which are risk factors for developing diabetic foot ulcers. This was confirmed in a study involving 33 people with type 2 diabetes who had developed foot ulcers. Compared with a similar group of 66 people who had type 2 diabetes but no foot ulcers, those with foot ulceration had significantly lower magnesium levels, and the people with the lowest magnesium levels were three times more likely to have a foot ulcer than those with the highest.[254]

Where you find it

Seafood, meat, eggs, dairy products, wholegrains, pulses, nuts and dark green, leafy vegetables are all rich in magnesium. Deficiencies are far from rare: one survey found that 80 per cent of American women following a typical Western diet had magnesium intakes below the recommended levels.[255]

More, it is one of the most common mineral deficiencies in people with type 2 diabetes. A Swiss study of 109 people with type 2 diabetes, for example, found they were more than three times as likely to have magnesium levels below the norm compared to 156 people without diabetes.[256] And as we've seen, the results can be serious. Not only is deficiency linked to insulin resistance, glucose intolerance and coronary heart disease; it's also implicated in an increased risk of retinopathy[257] and neuropathy.[258]

It remains unclear, however, why people with diabetes have low magnesium levels. Reduced magnesium absorption may be involved, but a study involving people with reasonably well-controlled type 2 diabetes found no significant difference in magnesium absorption and retention compared with non-diabetics.[259]

How much you need

The new EU RDA for magnesium is 375mg. People who are physically active may need more, as large amounts can be lost in sweat.

Side effects/safety

Intakes of up to 400mg a day are not associated with adverse effects. Some people do experience intestinal gas and loose stools when supplementing magnesium; magnesium gluconate is less likely to cause any of these side effects, although magnesium citrate is the most readily absorbed form. It's best to take magnesium supplements with food to optimise absorption.

Sodium and potassium

What they are

Sodium is a mineral found primarily in the fluid *outside* body cells, which it regulates and balances. In contrast, potassium is found primarily in the fluid *inside* your cells. The two work together via an electrical exchange to keep your nerves conducting and muscles contracting. In fact, the active transport of sodium and potassium ions in and out of cells is one of the main energy-using metabolic processes in your body. It is estimated to account for 33 per cent of the glucose used by all cells, and 70 per cent of the energy used by nerve cells. Potassium is also important for flushing excess sodium out of the body through the kidneys.

This section looks at sodium and potassium together as they work in tandem, and a balance between the two is important; but supplementing sodium is rarely necessary, given the amounts we get in our food. So the information on sodium here is primarily to do with *limiting* this mineral in the diet. (For practical advice on how best to do that, see page 90.)

How they can help or harm you

Sodium and blood pressure The high blood pressure that people with diabetes often develop is linked to the abnormal handling of sodium within the body generally, within cells and within the kidneys.[260] This may be due to increased sodium retention.[261] It has been found, for instance, that high blood levels of glucose and insulin both seem to stimulate sodium reabsorption from the filtered urine by the kidneys, thus increasing sodium retention. People with type 2 diabetes who have insulin resistance are most prone to this problem.[262,263] High glucose and insulin levels in people with type 2 also increase the loss of protein in your urine, which in turn boosts sodium and uric acid retention.[264]

The obvious way to remedy this problem would seem to be eating less salt. But the issue is not as simple as it appears. Some research has discovered that salt restriction in some people does not always have beneficial effects. In one study, an abundant sodium intake was found to improve glucose tolerance and insulin resistance in some people with diabetes who were salt-sensitive, or receiving drugs to treat high blood pressure.[265] Restricting salt in the diet has also been shown to lower insulin sensitivity in people with diabetes who had normal blood pressure.[266] These are odd findings. But we do not yet have a full understanding of how minerals interact in the body, and it could be that low levels of other minerals such as potassium, magnesium and calcium are behind these results.

On the whole, the consensus of opinion is that consuming too much sodium is harmful if you have diabetes. Blood pressure in people with type 1 diabetes is sodium sensitive,[267] and a relatively high sodium intake increases the chance of developing cardiovascular disease. The results can be rewarding – and swift. An analysis of 28 trials assessing realistic sodium reductions (equivalent to reductions of 4.66g salt/day) over at least four weeks showed blood pressure fell by an average of 4.96/2.73mmHg in those with hypertension and by 2.03/0.97mmHg in those with normal blood pressure in just that short time span.[268]

The Intersalt study,[269,270] which involved over 10,000 people aged 20 to 59 from 32 countries, suggested that the link between salt intake, and raised blood pressure linked to increasing age, is even stronger than previously thought. Higher levels of sodium in the urine were found to be associated with age-related high blood pressure, leading the researchers to recommend reducing high salt intake.

Some research[271] suggests that reducing your intake of salt by 3g per day (the UK daily average is 9g) can lower systolic blood pressure in people aged from 50 to 65 by 10mmHg, on average. Even better news is that this reduction in blood pressure is enough to reduce the risk of death by stroke at any age by 22 per cent, and death from heart disease by 16 per cent.

Potassium and blood pressure Potassium helps keep blood pressure low, so a diet low in potassium is linked with a higher risk of high blood pressure and stroke – especially if your diet is also high in sodium.

In one study[272] involving 54 people with well-controlled high blood pressure, one group followed a higher potassium diet while the other group kept to their normal diet. Over the following year, drug treatment was reduced gradually while always ensuring that blood pressure remained below 160/95mmHg. The potassium intake was checked monthly. At the end of the year, the average number of antihypertensive pills taken per day had shrunk by 69 per cent in those on the higher potassium diet, compared with 24 per cent in those on their normal diet. In fact, blood pressure could be controlled using less than half the initial drug treatment in 81 per cent of those following the higher potassium diet.

Where you find it

Food sources of sodium (mainly as sodium chloride) include table salt, salty snacks such as crisps and salted nuts, bacon, tinned products (especially those canned in brine), cured, smoked or pickled fish/meats and meat pastes, pâtés, ready-prepared meals, packet soups and sauces, stock cubes and yeast extracts.

Potassium-rich foods include seafood; fresh fruit, especially bananas, dried apricots, pears and tomatoes; fruit juices and fruit yoghurts; vegetables, especially mushrooms, potatoes, aubergines, peppers, squash and spinach; pulses such as peas and lima beans; wholegrains and breakfast cereals (check labels for sodium chloride content, as some may have high levels); and low-sodium, potassium-enriched salts.

How much you need

Sodium An average male weighing 70kg has around 225g salt in his body, and can maintain a healthy sodium balance with an intake of as little as 1.25g salt per day – as long as he does not sweat heavily. The UK RNI for sodium is 1600mg a day, but most people obtain much more than this, given the high amounts in so many processed foods. Ideally, an adult should obtain no more than 6g salt per day – around 1 level teaspoon. Target maximum intakes for children are proportionately smaller and were announced in May 2004 by the Food Standards Agency. (See pages

90–1 for more information on this, as well as ways of keeping your salt intake in check.)

Potassium There is no RDA for potassium, but it's advised to take around 3000 to 3500mg a day. It is estimated that 1 in 3 people get less than this and the average intake is around 3187mg. Some people obtain as little as 1700mg potassium from their food.

To increase your potassium intake, eat more:

- seafood
- fresh fruit
- vegetable juices (such as tomato)
- vegetables, especially mushrooms, potatoes, aubergines, peppers, squash and spinach
- pulses such as peas and lima beans.

Steam rather than boil vegetables to retain more of their mineral content. If you do cook them in water, make gravy or a low-fat sauce with it afterwards.

Side effects/safety

As we have seen, the main health problem linked with excess salt is high blood pressure, which in turn increases the risk of developing a heart attack, stroke or kidney failure. Excess salt has also been linked with health problems such as osteoporosis, fluid retention (equivalent to 1 to 2kg at some times of the month for women), asthma and even stomach cancer.

The rise in arterial blood pressure that occurs with age is, as we've seen, closely linked with high salt intake,[273] A high salt intake is also linked with thickening of the wall of the left ventricle of the heart[274], and with stiffening[275] and narrowing of the arteries,[276] which can happen independently of the high blood pressure. These changes, resulting from high body salt content, are due to an inability of the kidneys to excrete the large amounts of sodium chloride that we now consume.[277] So far, at least 20 genes have been identified that are associated with the development of hypertension and all are involved in the regulation of sodium by the kidneys.[278] Humans only began adding salt to their food around 10,000 years ago; we evolved and were genetically programmed over millions of years during which salt intakes were less than 1g per day. Native peoples with a salt intake below 3g per day do not show a rise in blood pressure with increasing age.[279]

Vanadium

What it is

Vanadium is a trace element whose exact biological function remains unclear, but may be linked to insulin and glucose balance, as well as growth and fat metabolism – low levels raise cholesterol and triglyceride levels. In the body it is mainly stored in the bones and teeth.

How it can help you

Vanadium may have a direct effect on diabetes. In 1899, the French physician B. Lyonnet showed that giving vanadium to people with diabetes greatly reduced the concentration of glucose in their urine (using the traditional taste test!). Modern research suggests it either mimics the effects of insulin or increases its action to improve glucose controls and lower insulin levels in both type 1 and type 2 diabetes.

Vanadium is also thought to help protect against coronary heart disease, lower cholesterol levels and have a beneficial effect on cholesterol and triglyceride metabolism, and help regulate the sodium-potassium exchange.

Glucose control In rats, vanadium has an effect that mimics insulin by helping to lower glucose levels and reverse artificially induced diabetes.[280,281] In humans, taking vanadium salts has also been shown to improve glucose concentrations by 20 per cent in people with type 2 diabetes,[282] and to improve glucose tolerance.[283] The beneficial effects of vanadium appeared to last at least four weeks after people stop taking it.

In one small trial[284] involving seven obese people with type 2 diabetes, glycosylated HbA1c fell by 6 per cent and fasting glucose levels fell by 14 per cent within three weeks. Similar effects did not occur in obese people without diabetes.

Vanadium may be effective not only in treating or relieving both types of diabetes, but also in preventing the onset of diabetes.[285] The mechanism remains unknown, although some suggest it may stimulate the breakdown of glucose, its transport into fat cells and its conversion into glycogen in the liver, as well as reduce the amount of new glucose produced in the liver. Vanadium may also act on insulin receptors in cells to reduce insulin resistance.

Interestingly, one study[286] found that people with type 2 diabetes had significantly higher levels of vanadium in their white blood cells compared with healthy controls.

Where you find it

Foods containing vanadium include parsley, black pepper, seafood (especially lobster and oysters), radishes, lettuce, wholegrains, sunflower seeds, soya beans, buckwheat, carrots and garlic.

How much you need

There is currently no RDA for vanadium, but 'A to Z' style vitamins and mineral supplements tend to contain around 10mcg. An average dietary intake is estimated at 10mcg to 2mg daily.

Side effects/safety

An excess of vanadium is toxic, and in some trials participants reported diarrhoea, abdominal cramps, flatulence and nausea when given doses of 50mg per day or more. Some studies have used doses over a thousand times higher than the amount normally found in the diet, however. The long-term effects of such high doses are not yet known, and they should be avoided.

Zinc

What it is

Zinc is an essential trace element needed for the proper function of over a hundred different enzymes. It helps to regulate gene activation and the synthesis of specific proteins in response to hormone triggers. It is vital for growth, sexual function, wound healing and immune function.

If you have diabetes, this will affect the way zinc works in your body. Raised glucose levels increase the loss of zinc in urine, and this can lead to zinc deficiency. As zinc has an antioxidant action, a deficiency may contribute to the oxidation damage that occurs in diabetes. Zinc is also important for the synthesis, storage and secretion of insulin, and a lack of zinc may affect the ability of the beta cells to produce and secrete insulin. This is especially evident in type 2 diabetes,[287] in which damage to the beta cells has been shown to contribute to the disturbance in zinc metabolism.[288]

How it can help you

Improving glucose control People with both type 1 and 2 diabetes tend to have low levels of zinc,[289,290] as the excessive urination that can happen with diabetes means a lot of zinc can be lost this way. Zinc has been shown to improve insulin production in beta cells within cell cultures, and to increase the binding of insulin to liver and fat cells.

A survey of 3575 people in India[291] found that among city dwellers, the prevalence of diabetes, glucose intolerance and coronary heart disease were significantly higher among those consuming less zinc. Raised blood pressure and triglyceride levels and lowered HDL cholesterol were also linked with a lower zinc intake. In another study, taking zinc supplements helped to lower glucose levels in people with type 1 diabetes.[292]

Not all the research tallies with this finding, however. A study of 30 people with type 2 diabetes found that more than 30 per cent of the subjects may have been zinc deficient. However, taking zinc supplements did not significantly improve HbA1c or glucose control, although it did improve their antioxidant status.[293]

In fact, overall, the relationship between diabetes, insulin and zinc remains unclear, with no obvious cause-and-effect relationships.[294] But as zinc has an important role in the synthesis, storage and secretion of insulin, the loss of it in urine is thought to make glucose control worse, especially in people with type 2 diabetes. Loss of its antioxidant action is probably also important in this context.

Healing foot ulcers Research suggests that leg ulcers are often associated with low zinc levels. So taking zinc, in addition to vitamins C and E, can damp down the inflammation and promote healing.

Where you find it

Red meat, seafood (especially oysters), offal, brewer's yeast, wholegrains, pulses, eggs and cheese are all rich sources of zinc.

How much you need

The new EU RDA for zinc is 10mg per day. Deficiencies are widespread: many people only obtain half the zinc RDA from their diet, and the older you get, the more likely you are to be deficient. Men are at particular risk. Every time a man ejaculates, he loses around 5mg zinc – a third of his daily requirement.

How will you know if you're deficient? One of the earliest symptoms of zinc deficiency is a loss of your sense of taste. You may also develop white marks on your fingernails (although this is controversial), oily skin and a loss of appetite, and get frequent infections.

Side effects/safety

High doses of zinc – 1 to 2g a day – can cause abdominal pain, nausea, vomiting, lethargy, anaemia and dizziness. A safe upper limit of 25mg per day has been suggested for long-term use. Zinc affects iron and copper uptake when taken at doses greater than 50mg a day.

Herbal medicines

I hope you are heartened by the sheer number of nutritional supplements that can help ease the task of balancing your blood sugar and insulin levels. But these are not all, by a long shot. We haven't yet touched on one of the richest sources of natural treatments for diabetes and diabetic complications: herbal medicine. Fortunately, there is a vast range of herbs, hailing from healing traditions round the world, that have special value in treating the array of conditions and body processes involved in diabetes.

Herbal medicine is an exciting area for people with diabetes as a number of remedies are helpful in improving glucose control and reducing risk of complications. In fact, many herbal medicines are as effective as prescribed drugs. It is therefore best to consult a medical herbalist to select those likely to be of most benefit to you, as everyone is different and has different requirements. Some herbs may only be available from a medical herbalist as they are not in mainstream use. It is also important to ensure that your glucose levels are checked regularly and that your dose of any prescribed drugs is changed as and when needed.

I cover a number of herbal remedies here, from prickly pear and aloe vera to ginseng and Gingko biloba. But there are many that have not yet been studied extensively, or even at all – so their efficacy might be backed by anecdote rather than laboratory tests. These include dandelion root, Jerusalem artichoke, jambul fruit, okra, guava juice, ginger root, liquorice root, juniper berries, salt bush, neem leaf, traditional Chinese herbal medicines such as *jiang tang san,* reishi, maitake, and fig-leaf, senna-leaf and even stringbean-pod tea. I mention these here only because you may have come across them in magazine or website articles. The fact that there are so many of these must give us hope, as it is likely to mean that more will be tested in future, and join the already impressive roster of safe, effective natural remedies for meeting the challenges of diabetes. In this chapter, however, I have looked in detail only at those herbal medicines for which there is a growing body of evidence suggesting they are beneficial for people with diabetes.

Below is a list of common conditions related to diabetes along with the herbal remedies that are most often prescribed to alleviate them:

- For glucose control: Aloe vera, bitter melon, fenugreek, garlic, ginseng, Gymnema, holy basil, prickly pear
- For diabetic skin ulcers: Aloe vera
- For eye health: bilberry, Ginkgo biloba
- To boost immunity against infections: Echinacea, Gymnema
- To improve cholesterol levels: fenugreek, garlic, prickly pear
- To lower blood pressure: garlic
- To improve circulation: Ginkgo biloba, garlic
- To improve erectile dysfunction: Ginkgo biloba, ginseng
- To reduce abnormal blood clotting: garlic, Ginkgo biloba.

Other herbal extracts that are mainly used for their antioxidant action, such as Pycnogenol®, are discussed in Chapter 8 on antioxidants.

The lowdown on herbal medicines

Power of synergy

In herbal medicine, different parts of the different plants are used – roots, stems, flowers, leaves, bark, sap, fruit or seeds – depending on which has the highest concentration of the active ingredient. Herbal remedies can have powerful effects, and as you'll know, many prescription drugs (between 30 and 40 per cent, in fact) are single chemicals derived from plant origins. Most herbal supplements, however, contain a number of substances from the original plant.

These have evolved together over the millennia to achieve a

synergistic balance which tends to have a gentler effect than pharmaceutical extracts, which typically contain only one or two ingredients. The risk of side effects with herbal remedies is therefore relatively low (see page 120, however, for potentially risky combinations of herbal preparations and drugs).

How they're prepared

Herbal extracts are prepared in ways designed to concentrate their active components. Tinctures are made by soaking herbs in an alcoholic base and may be described as, for example, a 1:10 extract, which means that 10 per cent of the tincture is made up of the herbal base, while 90 per cent is solvent.

Solid extracts are prepared by removing the solvent (such as alcohol), drying the residue and powdering it to make tablets or capsules. Solid extracts are described according to their concentration so that, for example, a 10:1 extract means that 10 parts crude herb was used to make one part of the extract. The more concentrated the extract, the stronger it is, theoretically, although more volatile components may have been lost, so the concentration does not accurately reflect its activity. Because of this, it is best to select a standardised preparation where possible.

Standardised extracts

The amount of active ingredient each plant contains varies, depending on a number of factors such as its genetic background, the soil in which it is grown, the time of year and methods of cultivation. As the quality of different batches of the raw herb can vary significantly, standardisation helps to ensure a consistent quality. It means that each batch you buy provides consistent amounts of one or more active ingredients and provides the same benefit. Although tests to determine this may only be done on one or two ingredients, this does not in any way discount the undoubtedly important synergy between the other components present, whose concentration has not been exactly determined.

One part of a standardised extract may be prepared from as much as 50 parts dried leaves or more, which is another reason why standardised extracts are so effective; cheap, non-standardised products may contain little, if any, active components. Standardised remedies are also more likely to be backed by reliable testing.

WARNING

Many herbs lower blood glucose levels. If you choose to take one of them, it's vital that you tell your doctor first. You will need to have your blood glucose levels monitored carefully, and may also need to reduce doses of certain medications beforehand. This must only be done under medical supervision. It is important that you continue to check your blood glucose levels regularly if you start taking a supplement, and that you are confident in adjusting your dose of medication as appropriate, according to your doctor's instructions. If your blood glucose control changes, let your doctor know.

Now let's take a look at the herbs that could join your array of natural methods for staying healthy.

Aloe vera

What it is

Aloe vera is a succulent with lance-shaped, fleshy leaves. There are over 200 different species, but only three or four are used medicinally, and the most useful of these is *Aloe vera barbadensis*.

Aloe vera juice can be made from fresh liquid extract (gel) or from powdered aloe. The fresh gel has to be stabilised within hours of harvesting to prevent oxidation and inactivation. When selecting a product, aim for one made from 100 per cent pure aloe vera. Its strength needs to be at least 40 per cent by volume to be effective and ideally approaching 95 to 100 per cent.

Traditionally, aloe has been taken internally to help a variety of intestinal problems, but is now also showing promise in controlling glucose levels. Externally, aloe gel is excellent for treating skin conditions – which makes it a boon for people dealing with diabetic ulcers.

How it can help you

Improving glucose control In a small study of five people with type 2 diabetes, taking half a teaspoonful of aloe vera gel a day for 4 to 14 weeks was found to reduce fasting glucose levels by around 45 per cent – quite a significant amount. The researchers concluded from this and other findings that aloe contain a blood glucose lowering agent, but its identity and mode of action remain unknown.[295]

Other trials involving people with type 2 diabetes who took aloe vera juice also showed significant reduction in glucose, as well as triglyceride levels, but this time within two weeks. This finding was backed by a recent analysis of 10 controlled clinical trials, which suggested that taking aloe vera orally might help lower blood glucose levels in people with diabetes, as well as having beneficial effects on blood fat levels.[296]

Healing diabetic ulcers In one test, human skin cells which play a part in wound healing were obtained from people with type 2 diabetes and healthy people, and cultured with or without aloe vera extracts. In the cells derived from people with diabetes, the aloe vera extracts were found to increase communication between them, as well as their growth, suggesting that aloe vera may be a valuable aid to wound healing in diabetics.[297]

Note, however, that aloe vera gel should not be applied to deep or infected wounds, as some evidence suggests it may increase the time taken for these to heal. Never apply aloe vera to an ulcer without the permission of your wound-cut specialist/nurse.

How much you need

If you want to take aloe vera orally, start with a small dose of gel (1 teaspoon) and work up to around 1 to 2 tablespoons per day to find the dose that suits you best. Aloe vera juice may be taken more liberally – 50 to 100ml three times daily.

Side effects/safety

As with most herbs, avoid taking aloe vera if you are pregnant or breastfeeding. It may contain chemicals known as anthraquinones, which can stimulate uterine contractions, and it also enters breast milk and may trigger stomach cramps and diarrhoea in infants. Some women taking aloe vera notice that it increases their menstrual flow.

Some aloe vera products contain a bitter 'latex' extracted from the inner yellow leaves of the plant. This has a powerful cathartic effect and taking too much will produce a brisk laxative response due to the presence of the anthraquinones. These stimulate the contraction of smooth muscle fibres lining the bowel and usually work within 8 to 12 hours. Of course, you might want a laxative effect, but it's important not to overdo it.

Many products claim to be free of anthraquinones, but independent laboratory tests on leading brands in the US found high levels of one of them, aloin, in juice when it was claimed to be aloin-free. Look for the International Aloe Science Council (IASC) certified seal, which shows the product has been produced according to recommended guidelines.

You may develop an allergic reaction to aloe, in the form of a mild itchy rash, when you apply it to the skin. Stop using it if this happens.

Bilberry (Vaccinium myrtillus)

What it is

The bilberry is a small deciduous shrub related to the blueberry, blackcurrant and grape. Bilberries are a rich source of anthocyanidins (also known as anthocyanosides) and flavonoid glycosides, chemicals that have important antioxidant and anti-inflammatory effects.

While the American blueberry has cream or white-coloured flesh, that of the bilberry is purple like its skin. We now know that bright colour in fruit and veg often signifies the presence of valuable nutrients and other beneficial substances, so this wealth of colour in the bilberry means its content of antioxidant pigments is considerably higher.

How it can help you

Bilberry contains a unique anthocyanoside called myrtillin, which helps to lower raised blood glucose levels.

Extracts of bilberry are used to strengthen blood vessels and the collagen-containing connective tissue that supports them, as well as improving circulation. Bilberry extracts are well established, too, as a treatment for many eye disorders, including macular degeneration, cataracts and diabetic retinopathy (all discussed in Chapter 2). Its benefits as a treatment for problems with vision arise from the antioxidant blue-red pigments it contains, which protect the membranes of light-sensitive and other cells in the eyes, reduce hardening and furring up of blood vessels, stabilise tear production, increase blood flow to the retina, and regenerate the light-sensitive pigment rhodopsin in the retina.

Bilberry extract's effect on blood vessels and connective tissues also aids vision. It appears to protect veins and arteries by stabilising the fatty structures that make up their inner walls, and to increase production of vascular structural compounds.[298]

Antioxidant activity Laboratory research has shown that bilberry extracts have a powerful antioxidant action that helps to protect LDL cholesterol particles from oxidation – an important benefit for people with diabetes, who need more antioxidants to stay healthy. The antioxidant action of bilberries may even outstrip that of vitamin C.[299]

Boosting eye health In one study, 40 patients (all but three of whom had diabetic retinopathy) took 160mg bilberry extract or a placebo twice a day for a month.[300] Those taking the placebo then began taking bilberry extract for one month. While taking the extract, 79 per cent of the participants with visible retinal abnormalities showed improvement, compared to none on the placebo. Similar results were found in a trial involving 31 people, of whom 20 had diabetic retinopathy.[301]

The antioxidant effect of bilberries may help to prevent the development and progression of cataracts, especially when combined with vitamin E. In one study[302] of 50 patients with age-related cataracts, bilberry extract plus vitamin E stopped cataracts progressing in 97 per cent of cases. Some researchers have also suggested that taking bilberry extracts can reduce short-sightedness, perhaps by improving the reactivity and focusing ability of the eye lens.

How much you need

Either take 20 to 60 of the dried ripe fruit daily, or 80 to 160mg of the dry extract (25 per cent anthocyanosides is best) three times a day. Those with diabetes may be advised to take more than this; as with other herbal preparations, only take under medical supervision.

Side effects/safety

No toxicity has been reported even at high doses, as it is water soluble and any excess is quickly excreted through the urine and bile.

Bitter melon (Momordica charantia)

What it is

Bitter melon, also known as balsam pear and, in Asia, as *karela*, is the unripened fruit of an Asian vine. It is used as a food (steamed or sautéed) and therapeutically in the ancient Indian system of ayurvedic medicine, as well as Chinese medicine, to improve glucose tolerance.

How it can help you

Improving glucose control The main active component of bitter melon, charantin, contains a mixture of steroid compounds that can reduce glucose levels. Most of its ability seems to be down to a chain of amino acids, known as polypeptide-p, found in the fruit, seeds, and other tissue of the melon.[303] This is believed to reduce or slow glucose absorption and lower production of glucose in the liver rather than affecting insulin levels. In fact, it appears to be structurally similar to animal insulin,[304] and the plant itself is often referred to as 'plant insulin'.

Studies so far have been small, and neither randomised nor double-blind. A small trial[305] involving nine people with type 2 diabetes found that taking 50ml bitter melon juice at the beginning of an oral glucose tolerance test significantly reduced blood glucose concentrations. When the melon itself was added to the diet on a daily basis for 8 to 11 weeks, this also improved glucose tolerance and glycosylated HbA1c levels. There was no increase in insulin levels.

In another trial,[306] single doses of bitter melon juice were also shown to have an immediate effect on glucose tolerance in some people with type 2 diabetes. An impressive 73 per cent of the participants developed significantly improved glucose tolerance.

The juice appears to be the most active form as one trial found that, compared to the juice, powdered fruit was ineffective.[307]

In a recent trial involving 100 people with type 2 diabetes, drinking a blend of water and bitter melon pulp produced significant reductions in both fasting glucose levels and in glucose levels two hours after a 75g glucose 'meal' in 86 per cent of the participants.[308]

How much you need

To help balance levels of glucose in the blood, take 50 to 100ml juice a day, under medical supervision only.

Side effects/safety

Bitter melon, in any form, must only be used with careful medical supervision and monitoring. According to one recent safety review, 'Adequately powered, randomized, placebo-controlled trials are needed to properly assess safety and efficacy before bitter melon can be routinely recommended.'[309]

Doses far above the recommended amount (see above) can cause abdominal pain and diarrhoea, and may affect enzyme levels in the liver. But the real risk of taking this remedy lies in its potential to cause hypoglycaemia (see page 49). For this reason, small children and people with frequent hypoglycaemia should not eat it. Reported side effects include hypoglycaemic coma and convulsions in children. It may also interact with other glucose-lowering agents.

People taking hypoglycaemic drugs should use bitter melon with caution, as it may increase the effectiveness of these drugs and trigger severe hypoglycaemia.

Coccinia indica

What it is

Coccinia indica is a creeper that grows wild in India.

How it can help you

Ayurvedic physicians have used it as an antidiabetic drug for centuries. In 1979, a small controlled trial was carried out on 32 people with type 2 diabetes. Ten out of the 16 taking *Coccinia* showed marked improvement in glucose tolerance, compared to none of the people taking a placebo[310]

In a more recent study,[311] dried *Coccinia* extract was given to 30 people with type 2 diabetes for six weeks, at doses of 500mg/kg body weight. The results led the researchers to suggest that *Coccinia* has an insulin-like action on enzymes involved in glucose metabolism.

How much you need

There is no known recommended dose.

Side effects/safety

Uncertain, so it should be used only under medical supervision.

Echinacea

What it is

Echinacea purpurea is an attractive flower also known as the purple coneflower, and is a traditional remedy first used by Native Americans.

How it can help you

It is known that people with diabetes can have suppressed immune systems and be more susceptible to infection with bacteria, fungi and viruses. So strengthening the body's interior defences should be an important priority – and taking Echinacea is an excellent way of doing that. Surveys suggest that Echinacea is among the most popular herbal remedies taken by people with diabetes, as it helps to reduce the risk of infection.

Echinacea contains several unique polysaccharides, or large carbohydrate molecules, known as echinacins that appear to stimulate immunity by increasing the number and activity of white blood cells. It especially stimulates phagocytosis – a process in which white blood cells gobble up bacteria and viruses before destroying them – as well as boosting the production of a natural antiviral substance called interferon. On top of all this, Echinacea contains flavonoids that have an antioxidant action.

Echinacea boosts immunity and promotes healing, and is now mainly used to help prevent and treat recurrent upper respiratory tract infections such as the common cold, laryngitis, tonsillitis, infections of the middle ear or sinusitis, viral infections such as herpes cold sores, and skin complaints. A tincture of Echinacea can be used as a mouthwash to treat and help to prevent recurrent oral thrush.

Fighting infections Echinacea has been shown to almost double the length of time between infections compared with those not taking it and, when infections do occur, they tend to be less severe. Most studies show it reduces susceptibility to colds by a quarter to a third.

A trial involving 282 healthy people aged 18 to 65 looked at the effect of starting Echinacea or a placebo at the first symptom of a cold – 10 doses the first day, then four doses per day for a week. A total of 128 of the participants contracted a common cold – 59 took Echinacea and 69 took placebo. The total daily symptom scores were found to be 23.1 per cent lower in the Echinacea group than in the placebo group.[312]

In another study, 259 people attending one of 15 doctors because they had caught an acute common cold either received Echinacea or a placebo 3 times a day for 7 to 9 days. Echinacea was found to be almost 21 per cent more effective at relieving symptoms than the placebo, producing a 34 per cent greater improvement in wellbeing. Benefits were noticeable by the second day and were significantly greater by the fourth day of treatment.[313]

Preventing candida One study found that in women with vaginal candida, combining oral Echinacea with an antifungal, econazole nitrate cream, reduced the rate of recurrence compared with those using the antifungal cream alone. As fungal skin infections are common in people with diabetes, this is worth being aware of.

How much you need

Choose products standardised to contain at least 3.5 per cent echinicosides. A good guideline is to take 300mg 3 times daily for colds and flu, or 200mg 3 or 4 times a day for lesser infections; but opinions on how to take it vary.

As it seems to work via phagocytosis – stimulating the activity of white blood cells that absorb viruses and bacteria before destroying them – and as this activity remains above normal for several days after a dose, taking it only during weekdays, and not at weekends, for example, or for two weeks out of four, should not reduce its effectiveness. The manufacturers of one of the leading Echinacea tinctures do not place any restriction on its long-term use, and say it may be taken in low doses over the long term to reduce infections, or in a higher dose just when you feel an infection coming on. Certainly there is no evidence of harm from taking it long term. Other manufacturers prefer their products to be used intermittently, say for no more than two weeks without a break.

Always follow manufacturers' guidelines on how to use their products, as some will contain a different balance of ingredients than others and should be used in a different way.

Echinacea can also be applied to the skin as a dilute solution to treat a variety of inflamatory and infectious skin conditions.

Side effects/safety

No serious side effects have been reported with Echinacea use. Some people develop a rash when using the herb.

Some Echinacea elixirs contain sugar – so check labels for sugar content, or choose tablets instead.

Fenugreek (Trigonella foenum-graecum)

What it is

Fenugreek, a strongly aromatic herb common in North Africa, the Mediterranean and India, has an antidiabetic action and the ability to lower cholesterol levels. Its seeds also have a wide number of traditional uses in ayurvedic and Chinese medicine.

How it can help you

Improving glucose control In one study, fenugreek seed powder (100g defatted seed extracts divided into two doses and cooked into chapattis) was added to a controlled diet for people with type 1 diabetes for 10 days. (The defatting process removes the bitterness.) Adding fenugreek significantly reduced fasting blood glucose levels and improved glucose tolerance compared with the same diet, except without fenugreek seed powder. The fenugreek group also showed a 54 per cent reduction in glucose excretion through the urine.[314] It was not clear whether this improvement resulted from reduced absorption or improved metabolism of glucose.

Taking 15g powdered fenugreek seed soaked in water was shown to significantly reduce blood glucose levels following a meal in people with type 2 diabetes. Insulin levels also tended to be lower.[315]

In another study, 25 people newly diagnosed with type 2 diabetes were randomly given either 1g daily of a fenugreek seed extract or a placebo for two months. At the end of the study, there was a significant improvement in glucose control and a reduction in insulin resistance in those taking fenugreek. Triglyceride levels decreased and HDL cholesterol also increased significantly.[316]

In one study,[317] 10 people with type 2 diabetes were studied for 30 days. In one 15-day period, 25g fenugreek seed powder was added to their diet, and in one it was left out. A glucose tolerance test at the end of each period showed that fenugreek powder significantly improved glucose control; it's possible that the powder's high soluble fibre content may reduce the absorption of glucose. An increase in insulin receptors was also found in their red blood cells. No side effects were noted.

Reducing cholesterol levels In people with type 1 diabetes, fenugreek seed powder was added to a controlled diet for 10 days. Fenugreek significantly reduced total cholesterol, LDL cholesterol and triglycerides levels, while HDL cholesterol levels remained unchanged.[318]

How much you need

Trials have used 15 to 100g defatted seed extracts, or 15 to 25g powdered whole seed extract per day.

Side effects/safety

Mild flatulence and diarrhoea have been reported as a side effect in 10 to 20 per cent of people using defatted extracts, but powdered whole seed seems to be well tolerated.

Do not take fenugreek during pregnancy.

There is a possible interaction with aspirin, warfarin and other blood-thinning drugs.

Allergic reactions have been reported.

Garlic (Allium sativum)

What it is

Garlic may be a popular culinary herb, but it also has renowned benefits for the circulation, as well as antibacterial and antioxidant properties.

How it can help you

The main beneficial substance in garlic is allicin (diallyl thiosulphinate), which gives the crushed clove its characteristic smell. Sulphur compounds formed by the degradation of allicin are also beneficial and are incorporated into long-chain fatty acid molecules to act as antioxidants.

Allicin prevents cells from taking up cholesterol, reduces cholesterol production in the liver and hastens the excretion of fatty acids, which in turn discourages atherosclerosis. Sulphur compounds formed by the degradation of allicin also act as antioxidants, protecting LDL cholesterol in the blood from oxidation and reducing their uptake by 'scavenger' cells to protect against atherosclerosis.

Improving glucose control Garlic has a weak blood glucose lowering effect and was found to improve glucose tolerance by 7 to 18 per cent in some early trials.[319] A recent analysis of randomised controlled trials lasting at least four weeks found no obvious effects on glucose tolerance one way or another, however, although many trials involved people without diabetes.[320]

Preventing coronary heart disease Clinical trials using standardised garlic extracts have shown that taking garlic regularly can reduce high blood pressure, lower levels of LDL cholesterol and triglycerides, reduce blood stickiness and improve the circulation. For instance, the extracts can lower blood pressure enough to reduce the risk of a stroke by up to 40 per cent,[321] and lower levels of harmful LDL cholesterol by up to 12 per cent, and triglycerides by 8 to 27 per cent.[322,323]

An important study focusing on 152 patients for over four years found that garlic tablets could reduce and even reverse atherosclerosis. In those not taking the garlic, the plaques that typically 'fur up' the arteries in atherosclerosis built up by 15.6 per cent over the four years, while the volume of plaques decreased by 2.6 per cent in the people taking garlic – adding up to a difference of 18.2 per cent.[324] Another interesting study found that garlic powder tablets can boost the aorta's flexibility, allowing the heart to have an easier time of it pumping blood out into the body.[325] Sulphur-containing compounds derived from garlic have been found to have a powerful antioxidant action that may reduce oxidation and glycosylation of circulating fats and proteins. This may have a beneficial, protective effect in people with diabetes and/or cardiovascular disease.[326]

How much you need

Select a product supplying a standardised amount of allicin (1000 to 1500mcg) daily.

Side effects/safety

Some people find the odour of garlic on the breath/sweat unpleasant. If you dislike it, select enteric-coated products.

Ginkgo biloba
....

What it is

Sometimes called the maidenhair tree, Gingko biloba is a very ancient tree species that has remained virtually unchanged for the last 200 million years. Its fan-shaped leaves contain a variety of unique substances known as ginkgolides and bilobalides.

How it can help you

Ginkgo extracts relax blood vessels and have a thinning action on blood, improving circulation to the limbs, hands, feet and head. By increasing blood flow to the brain, it improves memory and concentration and combats dizziness, tinnitus, migraine, dementia and some types of depression. As for the rest of the body, its boost to blood flow helps counteract chilblains, Raynaud's disease (where blood flow to fingers and toes can be temporarily interrupted, making them very cold) and impotence – which as we have seen (page 36) can be a significant problem for men with diabetes.

Improving glucose control In people with type 2 diabetes who are producing far less insulin from the beta cells than is normal, and who need to take oral hypoglycaemic drugs, it has been found that Gingko biloba can significantly boost the secretion of insulin.

Whether this happens because they 'resuscitate' exhausted beta cells, or stimulate the remaining active beta cells, isn't known. This effect was not enough, however, to reduce blood glucose levels during the oral glucose tolerance test, possibly because Ginkgo increases the breakdown of insulin and hypoglycaemic drugs within the liver. So if you take both Ginkgo and hypoglycaemic drugs, you will need to monitor blood glucose levels closely. This study[327] also found that Gingko reduced the level of circulating insulin in people who had insulin resistance and were taking oral hypoglycaemic drugs.

Reducing abnormal blood clotting Increased clotting due to clumping of cell fragments, or platelets, in the bloodstream increases the risk of cardiovascular disease in people with diabetes. Substances that thin the blood are therefore very important for diabetics. In one study, Ginkgo biloba as a potential blood-thinning agent was investigated in healthy volunteers and people with type 2 diabetes. Platelet clumping was assessed before and after taking 120mg of standardised Ginkgo biloba extract for three months. In the people with type 2 diabetes, the extract was found not to affect insulin levels, but did show a beneficial effect on platelet clumping.[328]

A previous study[329] involving 20 people with raised blood clotting factors and blood stickiness from a variety of conditions including diabetes, also showed significant thinning of the blood.

Improving problems with the eyes Ginkgo biloba's powerful antioxidant action and beneficial effect on peripheral blood flow make it a likely candidate to prevent or improve a number of eye conditions that people with diabetes are particularly vulnerable to, including glaucoma, cataracts, retinopathy and macular degeneration (see Chapter 2). And early laboratory studies have shown that Ginkgo has a powerful antioxidant effect in the eye that might be expected to help prevent diabetic retinopathy.[330]

Gingko has also been shown to improve visual impairment in people with diabetes. During this six-month trial[331] involving 29 people with early diabetic retinopathy, the researchers found significant improvements in blue-yellow colour differentiation in the people taking Gingko extract. This aspect of vision worsened in those on placebo.

Macular degeneration, where the part of the eye responsible for fine vision deteriorates, is a frequent cause of blindness. A double-blind trial[332] with 10 people that compared Ginkgo extracts with a placebo found a statistically significant improvement in long-distance visual acuity in those taking the extracts. In a larger trial[333] with 99 people who had macular degeneration, visual acuity was assessed after six months of treatment with either 240mg per day or 60mg per day of a Ginkgo biloba extract. The researchers saw a marked improvement in vision in both treatment groups after just four weeks, with a more pronounced improvement in those taking the higher dose. No serious side effects occurred.

Atherosclerosis of the carotid artery, which leads to the head, can restrict blood flow to the back of the eye – a condition known as chronic cerebral retinal insufficiency. In a study involving 24 people, the effects of Ginkgo biloba were assessed at two doses. In people taking 160mg a day, a significant increase in retinal sensitivity was observed within four weeks. In those on the lower dose of 80mg a day, this beneficial change did not occur, but happened only after increasing the dose to 160mg a day. Both doctors and patients noticed a significant improvement after the treatment. The results suggest that damage to the visual field in this condition is reversible.[334]

Helping peripheral vascular disease Ginkgo biloba extracts may be helpful as a treatment for peripheral claudication (calf pain on walking) that's due to poor blood flow to the legs. A pooled analysis of eight randomised, controlled clinical trials, published in 2000, found that taking Ginkgo biloba produced a significant increase in pain-free walking distance of around 34 metres – even in those using inclines rather than walking on the flat.[335] As the side effects are rare, mild, and transient, Ginkgo extracts are well worth considering (but check for interaction with other drugs such as aspirin and warfarin – see page 121).

Combating impotence In the laboratory, Ginkgo biloba extract has been shown to have a relaxant effect on the smooth muscle cells in the tissue of the penis,[336] which would be expected to allow more blood to flow into the area during an erection. Other studies have shown a dramatic difference for a significant number of participants, showing that Ginkgo can improve blood flow to the penis to strengthen and maintain an erection, producing a beneficial effect after 6 to 8 weeks in 60 men with erectile difficulties who had not responded to injections with papaverine, a muscle relaxant derived from opium. After six months, half the men taking Ginkgo had regained full potency, while another 20 per cent responded to the papaverine after the Ginkgo treatment.[337]

A study involving 50 males with impotence found that all those who had previously relied on drugs such as papaverine to get an erection regained their natural potency after taking Ginkgo for nine months.[338] In another trial, men taking 240mg of Ginkgo extracts a day for nine months experienced a significant improvement compared with those on a placebo.[339]

Improving mental function Type 2 diabetes can, at least indirectly, cause dementia because the increased risk of stroke means a greater risk of brain damage. Other aspects of poorly controlled diabetes, such as repeated periods of low blood sugar, can also harm the brain. Ginkgo biloba is emerging as a real hope, however, for improving memory and mental activity in older people. The most effective dose seems to be 120mg taken in the morning.

According to one review,[340] a number of clinical studies have shown that a standardised Ginkgo biloba extract is an effective therapy for so-called multi-infarct dementia, in which brain damage is caused by a series of small strokes; early-onset loss of memory; and mild to moderate cases of Alzheimer's disease. Ginkgo has been shown to improve a number of cognitive functions, such as memory, attention and alertness.

How much you need

For most purposes, take 120mg daily, either as one dose or divided into three. Select extracts standardised for at least 24 per cent ginkgolides. The effects may not be noticed until after 10 days of treatment, and may take up to 12 weeks to have a noticeable beneficial effect.

Side effects/safety

Mild headaches lasting for a day or two and mild upset stomach have been reported.

As with most herbs, it is best avoided during pregnancy and breast feeding.

A Cochrane review (produced by the non-profit healthcare review body, the Cochrane Collaboration) of the effects of Ginkgo biloba analysed all the published randomised controlled trials available. Their meta-analysis found no significant differences in side effects between Ginkgo and placebos. The conclusion was that Ginkgo biloba appears to be safe.[341]

Seek medical advice before taking Ginkgo if you are also taking blood-thinning treatment such as warfarin or aspirin, although at the usual therapeutic doses of Ginkgo, no effects on blood clotting have been found.

Do not use unprocessed Ginkgo leaves from garden trees, as these can cause allergic reactions.

Ginseng (*Panax ginseng*; *P. quinquefolium*)

What it is

Ginseng – usually referred to as Chinese, Korean or Asian Ginseng – is one of the oldest known herbal medicines, used in the East as a revitalising and life-enhancing tonic for over 4000 years. High-quality ginseng roots are collected in the autumn from plants that are five to six years old. White ginseng is produced from air-drying the root, while red ginseng (which is more potent and stimulating) is produced by steaming and then drying it. The closely related American ginseng (*P. quinquefolium*, which grows in the woodlands of the eastern and central US and Canada) has a similar action and is, in fact, generally preferred in Asia as it is sweeter tasting.

How it can help you

Ginseng contains at least 29 unique substances, known as ginsenosides, that make up 3 to 6 per cent of the dry root weight. Research suggests that American ginseng contains more of the calming and relaxing Rb1 ginsenosides, while Korean ginseng contains more of the stimulating Rg1 ginsenosides. Both, however, have been found to help with balancing glucose levels, and impotence.

Improving glucose control Ginseng is thought to lower blood glucose levels by stimulating the release of insulin[342] from the pancreas and by increasing the number of insulin receptors on cells – the spots where insulin can 'lock on' to a cell – to reduce insulin resistance. The main glucose lowering activity appears to be down to five other substances unique to ginseng, called panaxans, rather than the ginsenosides. It is therefore important not to select a highly concentrated extract (above 7 per cent ginsenosides), as this may not contain as many of the active panaxans.

In 1995, 36 people with newly diagnosed type 2 diabetes received either ginseng at doses of 100mg or 200mg daily, or a placebo, for eight weeks.[343] They were also encouraged to lose weight and to follow a diet supplying 30 per cent fat. All three groups lost weight, but the groups taking ginseng had improved mood, vigour, wellbeing and psychomotor performance, with the larger dose of ginseng also improving physical activity.

The people on ginseng experienced a reduced fasting blood glucose, with eight of them achieving a normal fasting blood glucose. There was little difference in effectiveness between the 100mg and 200mg doses regarding the blood glucose lowering effect, but the 200mg dose of ginseng improved levels of glycosylated HbA1c and physical activity. Overall, a third of the people taking ginseng achieved a blood glucose level within the normal range, with no change in blood insulin levels. This suggests that ginseng improves the insulin sensitivity of cells.

In 1999, an analysis of 16 well-controlled trials of ginseng root extract concluded that its efficacy is not yet established beyond reasonable doubt for any indication, including diabetes.[344] Yet other findings point to a definite effect on blood glucose, albeit one that is dependent on a careful balance with the consumption of carbohydrates.

In one trial in 2000,[345] 10 people without diabetes and 9 with type 2 diabetes were randomly given either 3g American ginseng or a placebo during 4 sessions, either 40 minutes before or at the same time as a 'meal' of 25g oral glucose. Their blood glucose levels were checked over the next 90 minutes, and those with diabetes were also checked two hours after the meal.

In those without diabetes, no differences were found in glucose levels after the meal when either placebo or ginseng were taken together with it, but when ginseng was taken 40 minutes before the meal, they experienced significantly reduced glucose levels. In the people with type 2 diabetes, significant reductions in glucose levels were seen with the ginseng, whatever time it was taken. The researchers concluded that, for non-diabetic people, it is important that American ginseng is taken with a meal to prevent unintended hypoglycaemia. In a similar trial involving people with type 2 diabetes, the authors suggested that no more than 3g American ginseng is needed to lower blood glucose levels[346] if people's glucose tolerance is abnormal.

Combating impotence Impotence is, as we have seen, a common complication in men with diabetes. Several studies suggest that ginseng can help treat impotence by increasing levels of nitric oxide (NO) in the spongy tissue of the penis. NO is a nerve communication chemical, or neurotransmitter, that is essential for – among other processes in the body – increasing blood flow to the penis during sexual arousal. Its action is similar in effect to that of Viagra.

In one interesting trial[347] with 90 men, the effects of ginseng were compared with a placebo and a prescription anti-anxiety drug (trazodone). During the course of the study, the three groups experienced no significant changes in how frequently they had sex, premature ejaculation or morning erections; but those taking ginseng were better able to maintain their erections and had healthier libidos and more satisfaction with the results, compared with the other groups.

In a recent study,[348] 45 men with impotence took either Korean red ginseng (900mg three times a day) or a placebo for eight weeks; the researchers then reversed what they received for another eight weeks. Sixty per cent of the men found that the ginseng improved their ability to develop and maintain an erection.

How much you need

With ginseng, the amount you take depends on the grade of the root. Work up from 200 to 1000mg standardised extracts (supplying 4 per cent to 7 per cent ginsenosides per day). An optimum dose is usually around 600mg a day. You can divide the dose in two, and take it morning and afternoon. If you have an entire root, you can take 1 to 2g of it a day.

Ginseng is not usually taken for more than six weeks without a break. In the East, it's taken in a two weeks on, two weeks off cycle. Some practitioners recommend taking it six weeks on, eight weeks off.

Select products standardised to contain around 7 per cent ginsenosides. This will generally be more expensive, but cheaper versions may contain very little of the active ingredients.

Side effects/safety

Caution is advised when taking ginseng on top of prescribed drugs, including warfarin, oral hypoglycaemic drugs, insulin and the anti-depressant phenelzine.[349] Always seek medical advice if you plan to mix medications and herbal remedies.

Ginseng is not advised if you have high blood pressure (it may make it worse) or an abnormal heart rhythm. Neither is it advised if you have an oestrogen-dependent condition such as pregnancy, or cancer of the breast, ovaries or uterus, as it contains oestrogenic compounds.

Side effects that have been reported with long-term use include sudden high blood pressure, diarrhoea, painful breasts, difficulty sleeping, nervousness, skin eruptions and euphoria. Together, these symptoms are known as 'ginseng abuse syndrome', but the people affected have reportedly taken 3g of the root daily for two years. High doses of 15g may cause feelings of depersonalisation and depression.

It is best to avoid taking other stimulants, such as caffeine (present in coffee, tea and chocolate), while taking ginseng.

When taken in appropriate amounts, as recommended above, in a two weeks on, two weeks off cycle, side effects should not be a problem. For those who find Chinese ginseng too stimulating, try American ginseng – it seems to have a gentler action.

Gymnema sylvestre

What it is

Gymnema is a woody vine used in ayurvedic medicine. Its Asian name, *gurmar*, means 'sugar destroyer' – an indication of its effect on high levels of glucose in the body.

How it can help you

Improving glucose control Gymnema seems to act in two ways to improve glucose control in people with metabolic syndrome or diabetes – by 'killing' sweet tastes and thereby helping curb poor eating habits, and by acting on glucose balance in the body.

When chewed or applied to the tongue, Gymnema reduces the ability to detect sweet sensations for up to 90 minutes.[350,351] It has been found to block the taste of sucrose, glucose and even artificial sweeteners such as saccharin and aspartame. So for people with diabetes who have a sweet tooth or want (rightly) to steer clear of artificial sweeteners, Gymnema could be a valuable herb to have around. Several unique, oily plant compounds known as saponins are believed to be responsible for the taste-blocking action.[352]

It has also been suggested that Gymnema may help regenerate beta cells. When given to healthy volunteers, it does not seem to affect blood glucose levels, but when given to people with type 1 or 2 diabetes, it improves glucose control and reduces the amount of hypoglycaemic medication needed.

In one trial, 200mg of the herb was given twice a day for at least six months to 27 people with type 1 diabetes who were also on insulin therapy.[353] A similar control group continued to use insulin alone. Gymnema was shown to reduce fasting blood glucose levels and glycosylated HbA1c. All those receiving Gymnema showed improved glucose control and had to reduce the amount of insulin they were taking to avoid developing hypoglycaemia during the trial. Cholesterol and triglyceride levels also improved with Gymnema treatment. The authors suggested that Gymnema enhanced insulin production in the body, possibly through action on remaining beta cells, as mentioned above.

In another trial, 22 people with type 2 diabetes were given 400mg of Gymnema extract a day, together with their usual hypoglycaemic drugs, for 18 to 20 weeks. Compared to a group using drugs alone, all showed improved glucose control. Significant reductions were seen in their blood glucose levels and most had to reduce their drug doses. Remarkably, five were able to stop their medication and maintain good glucose control using Gymnema extract alone. Significant falls were also seen in glycosylated HbA1c in those taking Gymnema. Just as with the trial mentioned above, the authors suggested that the herb may regenerate or improve the action of beta cells – a conjecture supported by the increase in blood insulin levels in those taking Gymnema.[354]

Acting as an antibiotic As people with diabetes can have lowered immune systems and are more vulnerable to pathogens, Gymnema's antibiotic properties – particularly against the common bacteria *Staphylococcus aureus* and *Escherichia coli* [355] – can make it a useful healing herb.

How much you need

Taking 200mg twice a day, or 400mg once a day, is a good general dose.

Side effects/safety

If you use Gymnema over the long term, you may reduce your body's ability to absorb iron, leading to iron-deficiency anaemia. As a result of this, a Gymnema extract called GS4, which has had components removed that are believed to interfere with iron absorption, is most often used in research.

No adverse effects were reported in trials where it was taken by some for 30 months.

If you do take it, monitor your blood glucose levels closely and adjust doses of medication as necessary, under medical supervision.

Gymnema may reduce appetite, and not just for sweet things. As with most herbs, it should not be used during pregnancy or breastfeeding.

Holy basil (Ocimum sanctum and Ocimum album)

What it is

Holy basil (also known, in Hindi, as *tulsi*) is a sweet culinary herb from India that is related to the European garden basil.

How it can help you

The herb is used in ayurvedic medicine to lower blood glucose levels, reduce high blood pressure and to relieve fevers, bronchitis, asthma, stress and mouth ulcers. It has anti-inflammatory properties.

Improving glucose control Holy basil is believed to increase the uptake of glucose by cells and to improve beta cell function and insulin secretion.

In one trial, 40 people with type 2 diabetes were given either holy basil leaves or a placebo (spinach) for eight weeks – all other diabetic medication was stopped. The holy basil was shown to reduce average fasting blood glucose levels by 17.6 per cent during the trial, and also significantly improved post-meal glucose levels.[356]

In another trial involving 27 people with type 2 diabetes, holy basil was said to lower blood glucose levels by 20 per cent, LDL cholesterol by 14 per cent and triglycerides by 16 per cent after 30 days.[357] The researchers suggested using the herb together with dietary or drug treatment in mild to moderate type 2 diabetes.

How much you need

The trials used 2.5g of fresh holy basil leaf in 200ml of water daily on an empty stomach early in the morning.

Side effects/safety

No adverse reactions were reported in trials.

Prickly pear (Opuntia robusta; O. streptacantha)

What it is

The prickly pear (*Opuntia robusta*) is both a traditional food among some southern Native American peoples, and a 'bush' treatment for diabetes. The stems (known as *nopal* in Spanish) may be broiled, diced and added to salad or tacos, or juiced. Prickly pear also has an antioxidant action.[358]

How it can help you

Improving glucose control Eight people with type 2 diabetes and six healthy volunteers took either one dose of 500g broiled prickly pear stems, two doses taken two hours apart, or a control. Blood glucose levels were then measured over the following six hours.

The healthy participants experienced no change in blood glucose after taking prickly pear. But there were significant reductions in blood glucose levels in the people taking two doses of prickly pear, with no big difference between those taking one or two doses.[359]

A similar study found that taking 500g of broiled prickly pear stems produced the biggest reduction in blood glucose levels three hours after ingestion.[360] Raw extracts did not produce a significant effect. The authors suggested that cooking may be necessary for the hypoglycaemic action to happen.

In another trial involving 24 people without diabetes who had raised levels of blood fats, both insulin and blood glucose levels were 11 per cent lower when they took prickly pear than when they didn't. The authors felt that prickly pear has potential as a treatment for metabolic syndrome.[361]

Lowering levels of blood fats Prickly pear contains pectin – a soluble fibre commonly known as a setting agent in jam-making. But pectin also has value in treating diabetes and its complications. It can slow carbohydrate and fat absorption, thus controlling the rise in glucose levels after a meal as well as reducing cholesterol levels.

A trial involving 24 people without diabetes who had raised blood fat levels showed that taking prickly pear for eight weeks lowered total cholesterol levels by 12 per cent, LDL cholesterol by 15 per cent and triglycerides by 12 per cent. The blood clotting factor, fibrinogen, was also reduced, by 11 per cent. All of this is obvious good news for people who have diabetes and are most at risk of developing heart disease or stroke.

How much you need

A sensible dose would be 500g of broiled stems a day.

Side effects/safety

Nopal is eaten widely throughout Mexico and in parts of the American Southwest, and no side effects have been reported.

12

Essential fatty acids

We took a fairly detailed look at dietary fats in Chapter 5, and discovered that the stars of this particular show are the omega fats – the aptly named *essential* fatty acids, or EFAs. This chapter looks in more detail at how EFAs can benefit you, if you have metabolic syndrome or diabetes.

EFAs, also known as polyunsaturated fatty acids, are divided up into two families: the omega-3s and omega-6s. Both are vital for our wellbeing. Quite a large chunk of our brain is composed of fats, for instance – some 60 per cent of its dry weight – and a significant portion of that is made up of EFAs. But there is much, much more. EFAs are also the building blocks of cell membranes, artery walls, sex hormones, and the hormone-like chemicals known as prostaglandins that are found in all your body tissues – as well as the sheaths surrounding the connections between your nerves. So they are an exceptionally important part of our inner landscape.

There are two main EFAs: linoleic acid (part of the omega-6 family) and linolenic acid (hailing from the omega-3 family). While your body can make small amounts of the EFAs from other dietary fats, they are often in short supply and must come from what we eat – nuts, seeds, green leafy vegetables, oily fish and wholegrains being the best sources. We get at least seven times more omega-6s than omega-3s in our modern Western diet, however, and therefore most of us have a relative deficiency of omega-3s.

When you don't get enough EFAs, your metabolism makes do with the next best fatty acids available. These might be saturated fats from meat and dairy products – but they won't have the same effect. They affect the quality of your cell membranes, the speed of communication between your nerve and brain cells, and may lead to dry skin, hormone imbalances and an increased tendency towards inflammatory reactions.

So it's important that you get the right kinds of fat in your diet – particularly if you have diabetes, because it is associated with a number of disturbances in EFA metabolism.[362] For instance, the body must metabolise linoleic acid (see above) to form the more active gamma-linolenic acid, or GLA, which is important in keeping down inflammation and the conditions associated with it, such as heart disease. But people with diabetes usually lack the enzyme activity necessary for the first steps of this process. So supplementing pre-formed GLA will circumvent the problem.

Most people with diabetes would benefit from taking omega-3 fish oils as they have such a useful protective effect on the heart, circulation and inflammation. As fish oils may affect glucose control, it is important to monitor your glucose levels carefully when first starting to take them. For those of you who are allergic to fish products, do not like them, or who are vegetarian, flaxseed oil or omega-3s derived from algae, are suitable alternatives.

Evening primrose oil helps to maintain healthy, supple skin and can improve the skin dryness that often affects older people. EPO may also be helpful for people with diabetic neuropathy. In addition, conjugated linoleic acid might help to reduce obesity and improve insulin sensitivity.

Below, I look at the essential fatty acids in detail.

Omega-3 fish oils

What they are

Omega-3 fish oils are extracted from the flesh of oily, coldwater fish such as salmon, herrings, sardines, pilchards and mackerel. They're particularly rich in the valuable EFAs known as EPA and DHA (see also page 77), which are derived from the micro-algae on which the fish feed.

Cod liver oil is derived only from the liver of cod. Compared to oils made from fatty coldwater fish, its omega-3 EFA content is only about a third as high, but this percentage can now be concentrated by processing. Cod liver oil also contains high amounts of vitamin A and vitamin D.

Regional and national studies suggest that people with the highest intakes of omega-3 fish oils have a lower incidence of diabetes.[363] A study in Norway has even suggested that giving infants cod liver oil during the first year of life significantly lowered the risk of the child developing type 1 diabetes, perhaps through its anti-inflammatory effects.[364]

How they can help you

Omega-3 fish oils help to balance the action of omega-6 oils such as those found in sunflower oil, which are mostly derived from vegetable sources. This is important, given the imbalance in the average Western diet in favour of omega-6s. Omega-3s are converted in the body to prostaglandins, which have a powerful anti-inflammatory action. Inflammation is now recognised as one of the main underlying problems leading to furring up of the arteries and coronary heart disease. It also contributes to the long-term complications of diabetes.

Improving glucose control The jury is still out over whether omega-3 fish oil supplements improve, or worsen, glucose control in people with diabetes. They have had a negative effect in some studies[365,366,367] and a positive one in others.[368,369,370,371] More recent evidence suggests that the effects of fish oil supplements on glucose control may relate to vitamin E levels. The 12 people in the study did not have diabetes, but the researchers found that when they took 30ml fish oil per day containing low levels of vitamin E (1.5 IU), their fasting blood glucose levels rose by 9 per cent. When taking fish oils with a higher level of vitamin E (4.5 IU), however, their blood glucose levels did not change significantly.[372] If you take a fish oil supplement, it is therefore important to ensure you have a good intake of vitamin E and other antioxidants. It is also vital to check your blood glucose levels regularly.

Another trial linked fish oil supplementation with exercise. In this, 49 people with type 2 diabetes and raised blood fat levels were divided into four groups. One group ate one fish meal per day and took part in moderate exercise, one group ate one fish meal per day and exercised lightly, while the other groups ate no fish and either exercised moderately or lightly for eight weeks. Blood cholesterol, triglyceride and glucose levels were assessed and the conclusion was that dietary fish can have a substantial, beneficial effect on blood fat levels in people with diabetes, but may have a negative effect on glucose control.[373] Moderate exercise seemed to improve the blood fat profile and offset the negative effect of fish on glucose control, suggesting that those who eat fish or take fish oil supplements should aim to exercise more.

A review of a number of studies[374] produced by the non-profit healthcare review body, the Cochrane Collaboration, was carried out in 2001 to determine the effects of fish oil supplementation on cholesterol levels and glucose control in people with type 2 diabetes. Eighteen randomised controlled trials were identified involving 823 people studied for an average of 12 weeks. The doses of fish oil used in these studies varied from 3 to 18g per day.

This Cochrane meta-analysis showed that fish oil can lower triglycerides significantly. LDL cholesterol levels rose slightly but no statistically significant effect was observed for fasting glucose, haemoglobin A1c, total or HDL cholesterol. No adverse effects were reported. The reviewers concluded that taking fish oil supplements lowers triglycerides and may raise LDL cholesterol, but has no significant effect on glucose control in people with type 2 diabetes, which is reassuring. Two previous analyses (one using the same data) reached similar conclusions.[375,376]

Improving cardiovascular health Omega-3 EFAs help to maintain a regular heartbeat and reduce blood viscosity, and play an important role in regulating blood pressure, cholesterol and (as we saw above) triglyceride levels – all of which can be beneficial for people with diabetes.

In one study, over 79,800 women aged 34 to 59 were followed up over 14 years, and it was found that women who ate fish one to three times a month were 7 per cent less likely to have a stroke than those eating fish less than once a month. Those eating fish five or more times a week had a total stroke risk reduction of 52 per cent.[377]

Another study looking at over 11,300 people who survived a

heart attack found that those receiving omega-3 supplements had a 15 per cent lower risk of death, non-fatal heart attack and stroke. This was attributable to a 20 per cent decrease in overall risk of death and a 30 per cent decrease in risk of cardiovascular death.[378]

Meanwhile, researchers analysing levels of omega-3 fatty acids in the cells of 291 people undergoing coronary angiography discovered significant beneficial correlations between levels of EPA and DHA with risk of sudden cardiac death.[379] A recent study[380] backed this up, suggesting that omega-3s significantly reduce the risk of sudden death due to arrhythmia after a heart attack in people with no previous cardiovascular disease.

Some heart research has also thrown up data on the effect, if any, of omega-3s on blood glucose levels (see above). For instance, one interesting study[381] involving 20 people with type 2 diabetes found that taking fish oils also had beneficial effects on the elasticity of artery walls without altering fasting blood glucose levels.

Another study looking at the blood-thinning properties of fish oil found that while blood stickiness and platelet clumping increased in five people with type 2 diabetes before they took fish oils, they decreased after eight weeks on fish oil treatment.[382]

In an eight-week trial looking at triglyceride levels,[383] people with type 2 diabetes took 20g fish oil per day, and halfway through, 15g pectin fibre was added to their regime. When taking fish oil alone, their triglyceride levels fell by 41 per cent and levels of VLDL cholesterol fell by 36 per cent. Total, LDL and HDL cholesterol showed no significant changes. When fibre was added to their fish oil regime, however, their total and LDL cholesterol fell significantly and their triglycerides decreased further by 44 per cent. Their diabetic glucose control stayed the same during the study. The authors concluded that upping fibre in the diet may increase the beneficial effects of fish oil supplements in people with type 2 diabetes.

How much you need

Taking 500mg to 4g daily is a good guideline for most conditions. For a severe inflammatory disease such as rheumatoid arthritis, up to 6g daily may be recommended. Cod liver oil is usually given in lower doses because of its high vitamin A content.

Side effects/safety

Taking fish oil supplements can cause belching and mild nausea. You can prevent this by shaking the oil with milk or juice to emulsify it – break it down into tiny suspended globules that will aid absorption and prevent 'fishy burps'. You can also buy ready-emulsified fish oil supplements.

Seek medical advice before taking fish oil if you have a blood clotting disorder or are taking a blood-thinning drug such as warfarin. If you are allergic to fish – a not uncommon allergy – you should avoid all fish oil products.

As we saw above, some research suggests fish oil increases blood sugar levels in people with diabetes but this is refuted in other trials. However, it also protects against the increased risk of coronary heart disease that can accompany diabetes. Taking high-dose vitamin E supplements along with them, and ensuring you stay active, have been shown to offset any rise in glucose levels, so if you do this while monitoring your blood carefully, you should keep the risks in balance.

Recently, the UK Food Standards Agency announced upper limits on oily fish consumption due to the presence of chemical pollutants such as dioxins. Women past childbearing age who do not intend having further pregnancies, and men and boys, can eat up to four portions of oily fish a week before the possible risks might outweigh the known health benefits. Girls and women who are pregnant, or intend to have children at some stage, should only eat between one and two portions of oily fish a week to limit any possible harmful effects on their future offspring. During pregnancy, it is important to avoid eating shark, marlin and swordfish and not to eat large amounts of tuna because of the mercury content of deep-sea fish.

Note that if you opt for cod liver oil, the ones labelled 'high' or 'extra high' strength provide the highest amount of omega-3 fatty acids. But if you take a multivitamin as well, check that the total amounts of vitamin A and D you are taking in both your multi and cod liver oil supplements do not exceed recommended doses. Vitamin A is best limited to less than 5000IU

(1500mcg) per day, although taking up to 10,000IU (3000mcg) is considered safe. The RDA for vitamin D is 5mcg (200IU), but those over 50 need to double this amount (10mcg = 400IU), as blood levels fall with increasing age.

Do not take cod liver oil products during pregnancy, as high amounts of vitamin A could potentially harm a developing baby.

Fish-free omega-3s

Given the importance of omega-3s to health, vegetarians and people allergic to fish might seem to be in a bit of a bind regarding supplementation. However, help is at hand in the form of flaxseed or linseed, pumpkin seeds, green leafy vegetables and walnuts (see below).

The cold-pressed dietary oil from flaxseed (not to be confused with the linseed oil used by artists and furniture makers, which is toxic) provides an omega-3 EFA, alpha-linolenic acid or ALA, that is a precursor to the EFAs found in fish oil. This means ALA must be converted by the body to make the more active DHA and EPA that are found fully formed in fish oil.

Taking flaxseed oil will provide you with an indirect source of valuable omega-3s. One to 2 tablespoons twice a day, preferably with food, has not been shown to have any unwanted side effects. Ensure that you store it in the fridge and don't use it past its sell-by date, as it can easily go rancid. Or you can eat the seeds, but you'll need to grind them – a spice grinder attachment on a blender will do.

It must be said, however, that so far there is no conclusive evidence that flaxseed has any effect on key conditions such as raised glucose levels, blood pressure or levels of blood fats. For that, we need to turn to walnuts – health in a nutshell.

Walnuts are not just a rich source of ALA. A number of trials have found that they help reduce high levels of blood cholesterol – which are a big risk with type 2 diabetes.

Analysis of five clinical trials involving around 200 people consistently found that eating walnuts lowered blood cholesterol when included in a heart-friendly diet. Those who added 84g walnuts to their diet every day for four weeks reduced their total blood cholesterol level by 12 per cent more than a control group. Harmful LDL cholesterol levels were reduced by 16 per cent.

Studies focusing on almonds and hazelnuts have also revealed beneficial effects on blood fats, and national and regional studies have also found a correlation between high nut consumption and a lower risk of coronary heart disease.

It is best to buy walnuts in the shell or in vacuum packs, as exposure to air rapidly reduces their nutrient value. If you eat 28g of walnuts a day (hardly difficult, as they're delicious), it would help to lower blood LDL cholesterol levels by 6 per cent. Will this make you fat? No: although walnuts are energy-rich (60g supplies 578 kcals), you won't gain weight from them as long as you eat them as a replacement food. Try scattering them over salads instead of bacon or cheese, chopping a few and adding them to porridge, or eating a small handful as a snack with an apple or pear.

Vegetarian DHA is also available from algae sources.

Evening primrose oil

What it is

Evening primrose oil is extracted from the seeds of the evening primrose oil plant. It is a rich source of the omega-6 EFA gamma-linolenic acid (GLA).

How it can help you

GLA helps to mediate inflammation, blood clotting, hormone balance and immune responses.

Preventing heart disease It was recently suggested that dietary supplementation with combined fish and plant-derived fatty acids such as evening primrose oil may be more effective in combating heart disease than taking fish oil supplements alone.[384] In this study, those receiving 4g fish oil plus 2g evening primrose oil were estimated to have a 43 per cent reduction in their risk of developing a heart attack over the next 10 years.

In another study, people with type 1 diabetes were divided into two groups. One was given 3g GLA mixture per day for two months. No changes were found in the control group, but improvements in beneficial HDL cholesterol and platelet stickiness were seen in those receiving the essential oil mix.[385]

Alleviating eczema/dry skin Many people with diabetes have dry, itchy skin, especially on their lower legs, which may be linked with essential fatty acid deficiency. A review of nine studies reported up to 1989 found that evening primrose oil frequently reduced the symptoms of dry itchy skin and eczema after several months of use, with the greatest improvement seen in reducing the level of itching.[386] Another study, in which adults with eczema received either 2, 4 or 6g evening primrose oil daily, and children took either 2 or 4g a day, saw significant improvement in the condition, especially at the higher intakes.[387]

Boosting metabolism of EFAs As we have seen, people with diabetes can have difficulty in metabolising EFAs. In an eight-month study[388] of 11 children with type 1 diabetes, supplements containing 45mg of GLA and 360mg of linoleic acid were compared with a placebo for their effect on EFA metabolism and prostaglandin levels. Their initial dose was 2 capsules daily for 4 months, followed by 4 capsules daily for 4 months. No change was seen with the 2-cap dose, but after taking 4 capsules daily, prostaglandin levels (which may lead to a reduction in inflammation) decreased significantly in the treated group compared with the placebo group. This suggests that the altered EFA and prostaglandin metabolism that occurs in diabetes can be reversed with evening primrose oil supplements, so that the body can make GLA more readily from linoleic acid. This effect remains uncertain, but if it does occur, it appears to take a while for benefits to show, and the dose of GLA taken may be important.

Alleviating diabetic neuropathy Neuropathy – damage to nerves, which can result in tingling or stinging sensations – is common in diabetes. One of the causes may be the abnormal metabolism of EFAs, as this is associated with a variety of vascular and clotting abnormalities that can lead to reduced blood flow and through this, less oxygen reaching the nerve cells.[389]

Twenty-two people with diabetic neuropathy were given either 360mg GLA or a placebo for six months. Compared with the placebo group, those taking GLA showed significant improvement in their neuropathic symptoms as well as how fast their nerves were able to conduct messages. The researchers concluded that GLA may have a useful role in preventing and treating diabetic neuropathy.[390]

In a larger trial[391] involving 111 people with diabetic neuropathy,

231

one group took 480mg GLA per day for one year while the other group took a placebo. Thirteen out of 16 different measures of nerve function significantly improved in those taking GLA over the year, but not with the placebo. The treatment response was greatest in those whose diabetic control was good.

How much you need

Taking 1 to 3g a day should be enough to see the beneficial effects.

Side effects/safety

The only people who should not take evening primrose oil are people allergic to it, and those with a rare disorder known as temporal lobe epilepsy, as it may make their condition worse. (although it has been used diagnostically to differentiate between this condition and schizophrenia).[392]

Conjugated linoleic acid

What it is

Conjugated linoleic acid or CLA has been much in the news lately. This fatty acid, mainly found in meat and dairy products, is being hailed as key to weight loss. And there seems to be some truth to the claim, according to the latest research.

CLA is formed in animals with more than one stomach, such as cows, by the action of an enzyme. It can also be produced commercially from sunflower, safflower and other oils.

CLA cannot be synthesised in the human body, and changes in farming practices, food processing and consumption of milk and high-fat foods mean that the amount of CLA we get has fallen by 80 per cent compared with our stone age ancestors. As a result, it is often referred to as the 'missing link' in weight loss management. Some researchers have even claimed that obesity is a CLA deficiency disease, as it is essential for the mobilisation and transport of dietary fats away from fatty tissues to muscle cells, where it is burned for fuel.

As an aid to weight loss, CLA is obviously important for people with metabolic syndrome or type 2 diabetes who are also grappling with obesity.

How it can help you

CLA appears to have an effect on the regulation of glucose and fatty acid uptake and metabolism. This may explain how CLA might help to reduce obesity, as well as improve insulin sensitivity.[393]

Helping with weight loss Intriguing research is revealing that CLA helps to promote a healthy body fat composition by increasing the breakdown of fatty tissue and the formation of lean body mass. It's thought to work by regulating the action of enzymes in fat cells so that less fat is laid down in them, and more is broken down and discharged from the cell, although the exact mechanism is not yet known. Once released, the fatty acids are transported to muscle cells to supply energy – thus building muscle at the expense of fat. Research has currently confirmed that CLA also reduces the size of fat cells.

In one study, 60 overweight or obese volunteers were divided into five groups and given a placebo or CLA in various doses every day for 12 weeks. It was found that those taking 3.4 and 6.8g of CLA lost more body fat, compared with those on the placebo. There were no significant changes in lean body mass, body mass index or blood fat levels, however.[394]

Metabolic syndrome and type 2 diabetes are, as we have learned, associated with abdominal or 'apple-shape' obesity, and some research suggests that dietary CLA may tackle this by helping to reduce waist size in obese males. In one study, 25 middle-aged men with metabolic syndrome and abdominal obesity received either CLA or a placebo every day. After four weeks, those taking CLA lost significantly more around their waist than those on the placebo. This suggests that CLA may help to decrease abdominal fat and needs further investigation.[395]

CLA's effect on insulin and glucose has also been investigated. In one of these studies, 64 per cent of people with diabetes showed improvements in insulin levels after taking CLA for eight weeks, with a moderately reduced blood fasting glucose level. They also had reduced triglyceride levels. This suggests that taking CLA may improve glycaemic control and triglyceride levels through improving the way the body handles glucose.

Lowering levels of blood fats One study looked at the effects of CLA in 51 people with normal blood fat levels who either took 3g of a 50:50 blend of CLA isomers, an 80:20 blend of CLA isomers or plain linoleic acid for eight weeks. Those taking the 50:50 CLA blend showed significant reductions in fasting triglyceride levels, while those taking the 80:20 blend showed significantly reduced VLDL cholesterol levels. There were no effects on LDL cholesterol, HDL cholesterol, body weight, plasma glucose or insulin concentrations.[396] This study suggests that CLA can have an effect on triglyceride and VLDL cholesterol levels – but that the blend used is important.

How much you need

Researchers estimated that the average diet supplies 100 to 300mcg CLA daily, while the most beneficial effects occur by taking around 3g daily. Trials have tended to use 3 to 6g daily, divided into two doses.

Products with a strength of at least 75 per cent CLA are most beneficial. Consider taking antioxidants with them to help protect them from oxidation.

Side effects/safety

Do not take during pregnancy, as its effects are unknown.

Putting it all together

Now that you have read the key research showing how certain dietary and lifestyle approaches can help you, and have looked at the evidence that many supplements are beneficial, it is time to work out your own, individualised personal care programme.

Step 1: Diet

First, you need to work out if you should lose any weight and, if so, how much. The optimum healthy weight range chart on page 55 will help you do this.

If you need to lose weight, you next need to decide whether to stick with the low-fat diet you may already be familiar with, or switch to the Atkins Nutritional Approach – the only low-carb diet backed by science. Information on how to follow the Atkins way of eating is available from one of the Atkins books (see page 99), and from the website (www.atkins.com/uk). Some people may prefer to follow a very low calorie diet under the supervision of a trained counsellor. More information on this is available from Cambridge Health & Weight Plan (www.cambridge-health-plan.co.uk).

If you are uncertain about following the Atkins approach, or if you do not need to lose much weight, if any, another option is to adopt a generally lower-carbohydrate intake by following a low-glycaemic diet – see page 68.

Step 2: Exercise

As well as following a weight-loss diet and considering lowering your carbohydrate intake, you need to work out an exercise plan that's right for you. You also need to increase your general level of day-to-day activity – tips to help you do this are provided on page 57.

Exercise should be an enjoyable part of your life that you look forward to every day. If you prefer exercising alone, choose:
• walking – especially brisk or hill walking
• cycling
• a home gym workout
• jogging
• gardening.

If you prefer companionable exercise, choose:
• walking a dog
• golf
• bowling
• table tennis
• joining an aerobics, keep-fit or dancing class
• tennis or badminton
• a rambling club
• a team sport such as netball, volleyball, ladies' football, rounders, cricket or hockey.

If you need motivation or someone to direct you, choose:
• a home exercise video
• an aerobics class
• a personal trainer
• an exercise class at a sports centre.

It is important that your chosen form of exercise fits into your daily routine, as this will make sticking with it more likely. This may be:
• early morning before setting off for work
• on your way to or from work (such as walking part of the way)
• in your lunch hour
• after work

- in the early evening – but only do light exercise (such as walking round the block with the dog) before going to bed, as otherwise it may interfere with sleep.

If you are unfit, start slowly and build up the time and effort you spend on exercise. Remember to:
- always warm up first with a few simple bends and stretches.
- cool down afterwards by walking slowly for a few minutes.
- wear loose clothing and proper footwear specifically designed for the job and use any recommended safety equipment.
- don't exercise straight after a heavy meal, after drinking alcohol or if you feel unwell.
- stop immediately if you feel dizzy, faint, unusually short of breath or develop chest pain.

Note that if you are taking medication, you must seek medical advice before starting a physical exercise programme. It is important to heed the warnings about avoiding a hypoglycaemic attack, and not exercising if your blood glucose levels are too high (see page 105).

Step 3: Supplements
....

Selecting the supplements that are right for you, as an individual, is not always easy. So consulting a nutritional therapist is money well spent.

You may already be seeing a dietician – a health professional who provides dietary advice for specific health problems such as diabetes or obesity. Dieticians are usually accessed through your doctor and, as they are classically trained to believe that you can get all the vitamins and minerals you need from your food, they may try to persuade you that supplements are unnecessary. I believe they are wrong – and this book covers a great deal of research supporting my belief, so they can investigate for themselves if they want to. Even government surveys show that few people obtain all the vitamins and minerals they need from their diet.

Because of this, I believe you would most benefit from seeing a nutritional therapist who is more fully versed in the benefits and potential dangers of taking vitamin, mineral and herbal supplements. Those with recognised experience, and who have professional indemnity insurance, are registered with the British Association of Nutritional Therapists; you can obtain a list by sending £2 plus a large (A4) SAE to BANT, 27 Old Gloucester Street, London WC1N 3XX. I am particularly impressed by the training offered by the Institute for Optimum Nutrition, whose members obtain the DipION qualification. A register of members (many of whom are also BANT registered) is available at www.ion.ac.uk; or you can find a therapist in your area by contacting ION, Blades Court, Deodar Road, London SW15 2NU (tel: 020 8877 9993).

As a basic, most people benefit from taking a multivitamin and mineral supplement (an 'A to Z' formula) plus an essential fatty acid supplement such as omega-3 fish oils. Depending on how well your blood glucose levels are controlled, you may then wish to add in a supplement, such as chromium, that helps to regulate blood sugar levels by improving insulin resistance in muscle cells, while conjugated linoleic acid (CLA) may help to improve insulin resistance in fat cells. Coenzyme-Q10 may help to improve beta cell function in the pancreas, while the antioxidant alpha-lipoic acid improves glucose uptake into muscle cells. Magnesium also seems to be important for glucose tolerance.

Antioxidants in general – including selenium, bilberry and pine-bark extracts – will help you because they have the potential to reduce the development of long-term complications such as retinopathy.

Garlic and Ginkgo biloba both help to improve circulation, and garlic also seems to provide important protection against coronary heart disease.

As each person's needs and medical problems are different, specific treatments to help specific problems (such as peripheral neuropathy) are best decided together with your nutritional therapist. You can also look up a particular problem in the index and turn to the indicated pages to read about particular supplements that are beneficial, if you wish to review your options.

A cautionary word . . .

As the following advice is so important, I make no apologies for repeating it again.

If you intend to make significant changes to your diet, and to take supplements, you do need to let your doctor know so they can guide you on how to check your blood glucose levels regularly. You need to monitor blood glucose levels carefully when starting to take a new supplement and discuss any changes in your glucose control with your GP. Only use supplements – especially herbal remedies – under the supervision of a medical herbalist or your doctor if you are already taking drugs to lower blood glucose levels; this is important to avoid hypoglycaemic attacks. Some supplements and dietary changes will reduce your need for medication so, if you are taking drugs, it is important that your doctor tells you how to adjust your doses accordingly.

Complementary approaches should always be used to support the medical treatment your doctor has recommended, and should never take the place of normal medical care. Never stop taking any prescribed medications except under the advice of your doctor.

Note also that the information in this book is not intended to apply to women who are pregnant.

Appendix 1

Exercise and type 2 diabetes: reducing the risk

Epidemiological studies suggest that regular exercise can play a role in keeping glucose tolerance balanced, and preventing type 2 diabetes.[397] And it is interesting that the protective effect appears to be strongest in those with the highest risk.[398]

The Finnish Diabetes Prevention Study, for instance, showed that changes in lifestyle, including exercise, of high-risk overweight subjects with impaired glucose tolerance reduced the risk of type 2 diabetes by 58 per cent over an average follow-up period of 3.2 years.[399] This was confirmed by the Diabetes Prevention Program, in which intensive lifestyle intervention also reduced the incidence of type 2 diabetes by 58 per cent.[400]

But how, precisely, does exercise reduce the risk of developing type 2 diabetes? Let's look at the possible reasons below.

The weight loss connection

Seventy-five per cent of the people who develop type 2 diabetes are overweight. Regular exercise will help you to maintain a healthy weight. Although the effect is small, it is particularly useful as a way of losing potbellies or 'apple-shape' fat round the middle. This kind of obesity is associated with insulin resistance, so it could follow that reducing waist size through exercise lessens this problem – and with it, the risk of going on to develop full-blown type 2 diabetes.

Glycaemic control

Weight training significantly lowers the response of insulin to a glucose challenge without affecting glucose tolerance. A meta-analysis of 14 trials showed exercise improves glycaemic control in people with type 2 diabetes, lowering HbA1c levels by 0.66 per cent, irrespective of any loss or gain of weight.[401] Although this may seem like a negligible change, research from Cambridge has shown that a single percentage point reduction in HbA1c levels can reduce the risk of having a heart attack, stroke or retinal bleed by as much as 10%. Similar improvements in glycaemic control are expected for people with abnormal glucose tolerance.[402] Older people who train vigorously on a regular basis have greater glucose tolerance and a lower insulin response to a rise in glucose than sedentary people of a similar age and weight.[403]

Intense, regular exercise and glucose tolerance

How intensely we exercise seems to be important in keeping insulin sensitivity up and glucose tolerance balanced. Low-intensity exercise, for instance, appears to be as effective as high-intensity exercise in enhancing insulin sensitivity in people with type-2 diabetes.[404]

Exercising regularly is also vital for such benefits to accrue. Among 14 older master athletes with a mean age of 61, for instance, 10 showed a deterioration in insulin sensitivity after 10 days' physical inactivity similar to that seen in young, lean, sedentary males. The comparable deterioration in the remaining four older athletes was serious enough to be classified as impaired glucose tolerance. Thus, a short-term effect of exercise seems to be normalisation of glucose tolerance.[405] Another study involving nine moderately trained middle-aged adults found that the beneficial effects of exercise on glucose tolerance only last for three days.[406] This suggests that you should exercise at least every three days.

242

Blood flow within muscles

Insulin resistance is associated with constriction in the blood vessels within skeletal muscle (muscle attached to the skeleton), which means that blood flow through exercising muscle will decrease. Exercise helps to overcome this problem, pumping up the blood flow through muscle while encouraging more blood glucose to move into muscle cells.[407]

Glucose uptake

The transport of glucose into skeletal muscle cells is mediated by an insulin-sensitive glucose transporter protein known as GLUT4, which is activated by two distinct signalling pathways: one stimulated by insulin, the other by contraction of the muscles during exercise.

As these signalling mechanisms are distinct, the maximal effects of insulin and exercise on glucose uptake are additive.[408] A single bout of exercise can promote glucose uptake into muscle cells even where insulin resistance is present.[409] Levels of GLUT4 increase with regular physical training and have been found to be around twice as high in trained men compared to sedentary ones.[410] Increased GLUT-4 concentration and recruitment may explain how exercise can reduce the chance of a person progressing from impaired glucose tolerance to type 2 diabetes.

Glucose phosphorylation and glycogenesis

Exercise improves insulin sensitivity by boosting the levels and activity of enzymes involved in glucose processing, and those involved in replenishing muscle glycogen stores.

Following exercise, glycogen – the storage form of glucose – in muscles is replenished in two phases, the second of which is insulin dependent, and diminished in people who have insulin resistance.[411] Exercise, however, can double the synthesis of glycogen during this phase because it increases insulin-stimulated glucose transport-phosphorylation.[412]

Muscle structure and insulin sensitivity

Exercise also improves insulin sensitivity through an adaptation in skeletal muscle cells. It increases the conversion of so-called 'fast twitch glycolytic' or IIB fibres to 'fast twitch oxidative' or IIA fibres, which have more capillaries and are more insulin-sensitive than the IIB kind – all changes associated with improved glucose tolerance.[413] Exercise has also been shown to increase the amount of polyunsaturated fats in the fatty membranes of muscle cells, which may also increase insulin sensitivity.[414]

Putting it into practice

How does all this translate into concrete advice for people who are at risk of developing type 2 diabetes?

First off, there is scope for variety, as both aerobic and resistance training improve insulin sensitivity. But the exercise must be regular, and you must keep it up: insulin sensitivity is greater in trained compared with untrained muscle, is enhanced by regular training, and is lost within days of inactivity.

How much should you do? The level of moderate-intensity exercise needed to prevent diabetes in 50 per cent of adults at risk ranges from at least 30 minutes per day to 150 minutes per week in various trials.[415] Glucose uptake is enhanced for up to two hours after exercise due to insulin-independent mechanisms, and a single bout of exercise can increase insulin sensitivity for at least 16 hours. There does not actually appear to be a threshold for the level of exercise needed, although excessive exercise which damages muscle has a negative effect on insulin sensitivity.[416] So don't become a gym addict. As with your diet, aim for balance – perhaps a regime that alternates aerobics with sensible resistance training.

Appendix 2

Weighing up anti-obesity drugs

If you are very overweight or obese, and have metabolic syndrome or have been diagnosed as at risk of developing type 2 diabetes, diet and exercise alone may help you get your weight within safe limits. It has been found that a weight loss equivalent to 5 per cent of body weight or more (usually around 4 to 8kg) has beneficial effects on blood fat levels, blood clotting, glucose control and insulin sensitivity.

But you and your doctor may find that for you, lifestyle changes alone may not be doing the job effectively enough. If this is the case, you may need help in the form of a prescribed anti-obesity drug such as orlistat or sibutramine. You will need to show that you're determined to lose weight, and that you have managed to lose a certain amount (see below) on your own.

Orlistat
....

Orlistat is licensed for use in people who are clinically obese (or who are overweight with other risk factors for coronary heart disease) and who have been able to lose more than 2.5kg in weight over a period of four weeks, using diet alone.

Unlike the slimming pills of yore, orlistat is not an appetite suppressant but a fat 'blocker'. It interferes with the action of a digestive enzyme called pancreatic lipase so that less dietary fat is digested and absorbed, and more fat is excreted through the bowel. Overall, orlistat (sold as Xenical) reduces the absorption of dietary fat by around 30 per cent.

Trials show that overweight people taking orlistat can lose nearly twice as much weight (and maintain that weight loss over two years) as those following a low-fat diet alone. Almost half of the people taking it maintain a weight loss above 10 per cent after one year. For someone weighing 100kg (15st 10lb), this represents a weight loss of 10kg (1stone 8lb) body fat – an amount that can significantly improve obesity-related conditions such as high blood pressure, abnormally raised blood fat levels and raised blood glucose levels.

Orlistat is taken up to three times a day – before, during or up to one hour after each main meal – and is prescribed together with a weight management programme that includes a low-fat diet. As very little drug is absorbed into the circulation, the side effects are mainly limited to an increased fat content in bowel movements, which may lead to feelings of urgency, flatulence and oily seepage. Other possible side effects with orlistat include: abdominal and rectal pain, headache, menstrual irregularity, anxiety, fatigue, hypersensitivity reactions and, rarely, hepatitis.

But there are also beneficial side effects. As one trial showed, by reducing obesity, orlistat also reduces total cholesterol levels by over 2 per cent, LDL cholesterol by an average 4.4 per cent, triglycerides by 23.7 per cent, systolic blood pressure by 7.9mmHg and fasting insulin levels by an average of 18.7 per cent after one year. After two years, 28.4 per cent of those in the treated group reverted to normal fasting insulin levels, compared with 16.7 per cent of those in the control group.

This is an important finding because raised insulin levels are a leading risk factor for the development and progression of type 2 diabetes. It's therefore heartening to note that only 4 per cent of those with impaired glucose tolerance at the start of three of the studies went on to develop type 2 diabetes, compared with 25 per cent of those with impaired glucose tolerance taking a placebo.

Orlistat has been shown to help prevent type 2 diabetes in the so-called Xendos trial.

The Xendos trial

The Xendos trial,[417] published in January 2004, was set up to investigate the long-term benefits of taking orlistat as a preventative against diabetes. (Xendos is an acronym for XENical in the prevention of Diabetes in Obese Subjects.)

Over 3305 obese people with a body mass index greater than $30kg/m^2$ were involved in the four-year study. Of these, 21 per cent had impaired glucose tolerance. All were given diet and lifestyle advice and half also received orlistat, while the other half received a placebo.

After four years, only 6 per cent of those taking orlistat had gone on to develop type 2 diabetes, compared with 9 per cent of those on placebo – with an overall risk reduction of 37 per cent. The difference in the incidence of diabetes was seen in the group with impaired glucose tolerance. So it seems that adding orlistat to a regime of lifestyle changes can reduce the risk of developing type 2 diabetes in people with impaired glucose tolerance.

This condition is, of course, often one of the symptoms of metabolic syndrome; and overall, 40 per cent of the people participating in the Xendos trial had at least three of the symptoms that define the syndrome. When the researchers looked at the data again, using just the results from people with metabolic syndrome, they found that those who had taken orlistat had:
- lost more than twice as much weight as those on diet alone (–6.4kg vs –2.9kg)
- a significantly greater reduction in waist size (–6.1cm vs –3.8cm)
- a significantly greater reduction in blood pressure (–5.4/ 3.1mmHg vs –3.5/2.0mmHg)
- a significantly greater reduction in triglyceride levels (–6.3 per cent vs –5.5 per cent)
- significantly lower rise in fasting glucose levels (0.08mmol/l vs 0.22mmol/l).

A similar increase in good HDL cholesterol of around 9 per cent was seen in both groups.

Moreover, significantly fewer people with metabolic syndrome who had taken orlistat, went on to develop type 2 diabetes compared to those on diet alone (9.8 per cent vs 13.7 per cent), with a relative risk reduction of 36 per cent.

Sibutramine

Sibutramine is a type of drug known as a monoamine oxidase inhibitor, and is related to antidepressants originally developed in the late 1980s. Sibutramine seems to act partly as an appetite suppressant, and partly by increasing levels of the neurotransmitter noradrenaline. Noradrenaline is related to the hormone adrenaline, and increases the body's metabolic rate by stimulating receptors in so-called 'brown' fat – a type of tissue that can generate more heat than normal body fat stores. It is thought that sibutramine may act on noradrenaline to increase the body's energy expenditure.

Researchers have found that people taking a low dose of sibutramine lost an extra 1.5kg of body weight over an eight-week period, compared to people not taking the drug, while those on a higher dose lost an additional 3.5kg/day compared with those taking a placebo over the same period.

In trials with sibutramine, 90 per cent of people who responded during the first four weeks of treatment went on to lose 7.7kg by the end of a year. In comparison, of the people taking a placebo, only 61 per cent managed to lose 2.4kg after 12 months' treatment.

There are possible side effects with sibutramine, however, including raised blood pressure, irritability and insomnia. Some studies showed a rise in average heart rate of four to six beats per minute, and an increase in average blood pressure of 1 to 4mm Hg. This is linked to the increased metabolic rate. Other possible side effects with sibutramine include: constipation, dry mouth, nausea, taste disturbances, diarrhoea, vomiting, palpitations, flushing, light-headedness, pins and needles, headache, depression, seizures, sexual dysfunction, menstrual disturbances, urinary retention, low platelet count, blurred vision, hypersensitivity reactions and kidney problems.

Appendix 3

Low-carb diets and diabetic conditions

There is a great deal of controversy over which diet is the most effective for people with type 2 diabetes. We touched on this in Chapter 6, and I am personally convinced that a controlled carbohydrate programme such as that pioneered by the late Dr Robert Atkins is the safest option to both prevent and control metabolic syndrome and type 2 diabetes.

A large body of evidence is accumulating that, I suspect, will slowly convince more and more healthcare professionals that people with poor glycaemic control will benefit from eating less carbohydrate. Some of the more compelling studies are covered below, to provide background information for those who want to explore further. A new book, *The Atkins Diabetes Revolution* (Thorsons), is a comprehensive treatment of the Atkins approach vis-à-vis diabetes.

Journal of the American College of Nutrition

One study from 1998 showed that following a low-carbohydrate diet can significantly improve glucose control. Twenty-eight people with type 2 diabetes who could not achieve good glucose control on their current treatment participated.[418] Of these, 9 were previously being treated via diet alone, while 19 were on oral drugs to lower blood glucose levels (although these were discontinued at the start of the trial).

The volunteers were put on a diet based on their ideal body

weight, and supplying only 25 per cent of daily energy in the form of carbohydrate. After eight weeks, the participants were switched onto a diet that provided the same amount of energy, but supplied 55 per cent carbohydrate – the conventional recommendation for a 'healthy' diet.

It was found that after the first eight low-carb weeks, the volunteers showed significant improvements in blood glucose control as shown by fasting blood glucose levels and HbA1c levels (see page 48). The people who had stopped taking their oral glucose-lowering medication also showed significant reductions in their weight and blood pressure. However, when the participants switched to the 55 per cent carbohydrate diet, their glucose control worsened again and their HbA1c level rose significantly over the following 12 weeks.

The study concluded that a low-carbohydrate, low-calorie diet had beneficial effects in people with type 2 diabetes who had failed to improve on diet or drug treatment alone, and that the low-carb approach may reduce the need to move on to insulin treatment.

American Heart Association
....

Researchers funded by the American Heart Association[419] randomised 53 obese females to follow either a very low-carbohydrate diet or a calorie-restricted, low-fat diet for six months. Both groups reduced their calorie intake by similar amounts (from 1608 to 1302 kcals daily for the low-carb group, and from 1707 to 1247 kcals for the low-fat group) even though those on the low-carbohydrate diet were told they could eat all they wanted as long as it was low-carb.

Although both groups consumed similar amounts of calories, the low-carb group lost both more weight (8.5kg vs 3.9kg) and more body fat (4.8kg vs 2kg) than the low-fat group, with no harmful effects on heart disease risk factors. At six months, the intake of saturated fat for the low-carb diet group was not excessive (20.7 per cent) and they had significantly increased their intakes of beneficial monounsaturated fat to 20.6 per cent energy intake, and of polyunsaturated fat to 9 per cent. (Monounsaturated fats include olive and rapeseed oils; polyunsaturated fats, fish and flaxseed oils. It has been found that these fats have significant beneficial effects on risk factors for coronary heart disease.)

So, even through the low-carb dieters ate more calories per day by six months compared with those on the low-fat diet, they lost significantly more weight and more body fat. This trial, and others, suggest that following a low-carbohydrate diet provides a metabolic advantage. In fact, the authors state:

> For the greater weight loss in the low-carbohydrate diet to result from decreased calorie consumption alone, the group would have had to consume 300 fewer calories per day over the first 3 months compared with the low-fat diet group.... Although the inaccuracy of dietary records for obese subjects is well documented, it seems unlikely that a systematic discrepancy of this magnitude occurred between groups of subjects who were comparably overweight.

As well as concluding that a very low-carbohydrate diet was more effective than a low-fat diet for short-term weight loss, the authors also concluded that a very low-carbohydrate diet was not associated with harmful effects on important cardiovascular risk factors in healthy women.

New England Journal of Medicine

Two other important studies were published during 2003 in the *New England Journal of Medicine*.

One involved 63 obese men and women who had an average body mass index of $34kg/m^2$. Volunteers were randomised to follow either a low-carbohydrate (and therefore high-protein, high-fat) diet, or a conventional calorie-restricted, low-fat diet. During the trial, professional contact was minimal as the researchers aimed to replicate the approach used by most dieters, who have to go it alone.

Those on the low-carbohydrate diet had a statistically significant greater weight loss for the first six months (7 per cent body weight versus 3.2 per cent body weight) and maintained a greater weight loss at 12 months (even though their carbohydrate intake had been increased).[420] Both diets significantly decreased diastolic blood pressure and the insulin response to a known intake of glucose. There was little difference in the LDL cholesterol between the two groups but, importantly, those on the low-carbohydrate diet showed greater improvements in their triglyceride and HDL cholesterol levels than those on the conventional low-fat diet.

In fact, these beneficial changes were as good as can be obtained with some medications and the researchers concluded: 'The low-carbohydrate diet was associated with a greater improvement in some risk factors for coronary heart disease' and also stated that '. . . the changes are greater than those expected from a moderate weight loss alone'.

The other trial involved 132 severely obese men and women with an average body mass index of 43kg/m2, randomly assigned to follow either a low-carbohydrate diet or a conventional calorie-restricted, low-fat diet for six months. Thirty-nine per cent had diabetes; of the rest, 43 per cent were diagnosed as having meta-bolic syndrome. Overall, 79 volunteers completed the study, with those following the low-fat diet being twice as likely to drop out as those on the low-carb diet.

The people following the low-carb diet lost more weight than those on the low-fat diet (5.8kg vs 1.9kg), whether or not they were using drugs to lower their blood glucose or cholesterol levels.[421] Nine out of the 64 people starting the low-carbohydrate diet eventually lost at least 10 per cent of their starting body weight, compared with only 2 out of the 68 people who started on the low-fat diet. For those on the low-carb diet, triglyceride levels fell by over 20 per cent; for those on the low-fat diet, the comparable figure was only 4 per cent. Insulin sensitivity was measured in the people with diabetes and was found to have improved more in those following the low-carbohydrate diet. In fact, the authors concluded that being assigned to the low-carbo-hydrate diet was an independent predictor for improvements in triglyceride levels and insulin sensitivity.

These same patients were followed up one year later and reassessed.[422] Those in the low-carbohydrate group continued to show more favourable levels of triglycerides and HDL cholesterol than those on the low-fat diet, and glucose control in those with diabetes or metabolic syndrome (as shown by HbA1c levels) on the low-carb diet continued to show significant improvements. Other metabolic factors were similar in both groups, but the researchers concluded that: 'Participants on a low-carb diet had more favourable overall outcomes at 1 year than did those on a conventional diet.' They also stated: 'Weight loss was similar between groups, but effects on atherogenic dyslipidaemia [raised triglycerides, lowered LDL cholesterol and proliferation of dense HDL cholesterol particles] and glycemic control were still more favourable with a low-carb diet after adjustment for differences in weight loss.'

American Journal of Medicine

A trial investigating the effect of a low-carbohydrate programme on blood fat levels[423] was published in the *American Journal of Medicine* in 2004.

In it, 51 overweight or obese volunteers were placed on a diet providing 25g carbohydrate or less for six months. Exercise recommendations, nutritional supplements and group meetings were given as support and 80 per cent of participants successfully completed the study. After six months, they had lost an average 10.3 per cent of their body weight. Their total cholesterol levels decreased by 11mg/dl (0.28 mmol/l), LDL cholesterol decreased by 10mg/dl (0.26mmol/l), and triglycerides decreased by 56mg/dl (0.63mmol/l).

Annals of Internal Medicine

An important study[424] published in 2004 involved 120 obese people with high total cholesterol, LDL cholesterol and/or raised triglycerides.

They were randomised to follow either a low-carbohydrate or a traditional low-fat diet. It was found that participants were twice as likely to drop out if they were following a low-fat diet. For those on the low-carb diet, the average weight loss was 12kg, compared to 6.5kg for those following the low-fat diet. The low-carb group showed more beneficial changes in triglyceride levels (a reduction of 0.84 mmol/l vs a reduction 0.31 mmol/l) and HDL cholesterol (increased by 0.14 mmol/l vs a decrease of 0.04 mmol/l) than the low-fat group. There were no statistically significant differences in LDL cholesterol, and the authors concluded: 'During active weight loss, serum triglyceride levels decreased more, and HDL cholesterol increased more with the low-carb diet than with the low-fat diet.'

Notes

INTRODUCTION
1   McCarty, MF. 2000. Toward a wholly nutritional therapy for type 2 diabetes. *Med Hypotheses.* 54;3:483–7.
2   Yeh, GY *et al.* 2003. Systematic review of herbs and dietary supplements for glycemic control in diabetes. *Diabetes Care.* 26;4:1277–94.
3   Ryan, EA, Pick, ME, Marceau, C. 2001. Use of alternative medicines in diabetes mellitus. *Diabet Med.* 18;3:242–5.

CHAPTER 3
4   Desouza, C *et al.* 2002. Drugs affecting homocysteine metabolism: Impact on cardiovascular risk. *Drugs.* 62;4:605–16.
5   Wulffele, MG *et al.* 2003. Effects of short-term treatment with metformin on serum concentrations of homocysteine, folate and vitamin B12 in type 2 diabetes mellitus: A randomized, placebo-controlled trial. *J Intern Med.* 254;5:455–63.
6   Armand, ASK, Carlson, SM. 1998. Folate administration reduces circulating homocysteine levels in MIDDY patients on long-term metformin treatment. *J Intern Med.* 244;2:169–74.

CHAPTER 4
7   McKinney, PA *et al.* 1999. Perinatal and neonatal determinants of childhood type 1 diabetes: A case-control study in Yorkshire, UK. *Diabetes Care.* 22;6:928–32.
8   Verge, CF *et al.* 1994. Environmental factors in childhood IDDM: A population-based, case-control study. *Diabetes Care.* 17;12:1381–9.
9   Hypponen, E *et al.* 2001. Intake of vitamin D and risk of type 1 diabetes: A birth-cohort study. *Lancet.* 358(9292):1500–3.

CHAPTER 6

10 Pirozzo, S *et al.* 2004. Advice on low-fat diets for obesity (Cochrane Review) in *The Cochrane Library*, issue 1. Chichester, UK: John Wiley & Sons Ltd.

11 Ginsberg, JH *et al.* 1976. Induction of hypertriglyceridemia by a low-fat diet. *J Clin Endocrinol Metab* 12:729–735.

12 Coulston, AM *et al.* 1989. Persistence of hypertriglycerolemic effect of low-fat high-carbohydrate diets in NIDDM patients. *Diabetes Care* 12:94–101.

13 Garg, A *et al.* 1994. Effects of varying carbohydrate content of diet in patients with non-insulin-dependent diabetes mellitus. *JAMA.* 271:1421–1428.

14 Garg, A *et al.* 1994. Effects of varying carbohydrate content of diet win patients with non-insulin-dependent diabetes mellitus. *JAMA.* 271:1421–1428.

15 Garg, A. 1998. High-monounsaturated-fat diets for patients with diabetes mellitus: A meta-analysis. *Am J Clin Nutr.* 67 (suppl): 577S–582S.

16 Liu, S *et al.* 2000. A prospective study of dietary glycemic load, carbohydrate intake, and risk of coronary heart disease in US women. *Am J Clin Nutr.* 71;6:1455–61.

CHAPTER 7

17 Adapted from: Health Supplements Information Service analysis of the National Diet and Nutrition Survey 2003.

18 Fletcher, RH, Fairfield, KM. 2002. Vitamins for chronic disease prevention in adults: Clinical applications. *JAMA* 287:3127–3129.

19 Rimm, EB *et al.* 1998. Folate and vitamin B6 from diet and supplements in relation to risk of coronary heart disease among women. *JAMA* 279;5:359–64.

20 Barringer, TA *et al.* 2003. Effect of a multivitamin and mineral supplement on infection and quality of life: A randomised double-blind, placebo-controlled trial. *Ann Intern Med* 138:365–371.

21 Leske, MC *et al.* 1991. The lens opacities case-control study: Risk factors for cataract. *Arch Ophthalmol.* 109;2:244–51.

CHAPTER 8

22 Borcea, V *et al.* 1999. Alpha-lipoic acid decreases oxidative stress even in diabetic patients with poor glycemic control and albu-minuria. *Free Radic Biol Med.* Jun; 26(11–12):1495–500.

23 Jacob, S *et al.* 1995. Enhancement of glucose disposal in patients with type 2 diabetes by alpha-lipoic acid. *Arzneimittel-Forschung*, 45:872–4.

24 Jacob, S *et al.* 1999. Oral administration of RAC-alpha-lipoic acid modulates insulin sensitivity in patients with type-2 diabetes mellitus: a placebo-controlled pilot trial. *Free Radic Biol Med.* 27;3–4:309–14.

25 Androne, L *et al.* 2000. In vivo effect of lipoic acid on lipid peroxidation in patients with diabetic neuropathy. *In Vivo.* 14;2:327–30.

26 Haak, E *et al.* 2000. Effects of alpha-lipoic acid on microcirculation in patients with peripheral diabetic neuropathy. *Exp Clin Endocrinol Diabetes.* 108;3:168–74.

27 Ametov, AS *et al.* 2003. The sensory symptoms of diabetic polyneuropathy are improved with alpha-lipoic acid: The SYDNEY trial. *Diabetes Care.* 26;3:770–6.

28 Ziegler D, Gries FA, Alpha-lipoic acid in the treatment of diabetic peripheral and cardiac autonomic neuropathy. *Diabetes,* 1997; 46:Suppl. 2:S62–6.

29 Ruhnau, KJ *et al.* 1999. Effects of 3–week oral treatment with the antioxidant thioctic acid (alpha-lipoic acid) in symptomatic diabetic polyneuropathy. *Diabet Med.* 16;12:1040–3.

30 Ziegler, D *et al.* 1999. Alpha-lipoic acid in the treatment of diabetic polyneuropathy in Germany: Current evidence from clinical trials. *Exp Clin Endocrinol Diabetes.* 107;7:421–30.

31 Morcos, M *et al.* 2001. Effect of alpha-lipoic acid on the progression of endothelial cell damage and albuminuria in patients with diabetes mellitus: An exploratory study. *Diabetes Res Clin Pract.* 52;3:175–83.

32 Facchini, F *et al.* 1996. Relation between dietary vitamin intake and resistance to insulin-mediated glucose disposal in healthy volunteers. *Am J Clin Nutr* 63:946–9.

33 Suzuki, K *et al.* 2002. Relationship between serum carotenoids and hyperglycemia: a population-based cross-sectional study. *J Epidemiol.* 12;5:357–66.

34 Ylonen, K *et al.* 2003. Dietary intakes and plasma concentrations of carotenoids and tocopherols in relation to glucose metabolism in subjects at high risk of type 2 diabetes: The Botnia Dietary Study. *Am J Clin Nutr.* 77;6:1434–41.

35 Baena, RM *et al.* 2002. Vitamin A, retinol binding protein and lipids in type 1 diabetes mellitus. *Eur J Clin Nutr.* 56;1:44–50.

36 Pauleikhoff, D, van Kuijk, FJ, Bird, AC. 2001. Macular pigment

257

and age-related macular degeneration. *Der Ophthalmologe.* Jun 98 (6), p511–9.

37 Junghans, A, Sies, H, Stahl, W. 2001. Macular pigments lutein and zeaxanthin as blue light filters studied in liposomes. *Arch Biochem Biophys* 15 Jul, 391 (2), p160–4.

38 Bone, RA *et al.* 2001. Macular pigment in donor eyes with and without AMD: A case-control study. *Invest Ophthal Vis Sci.* 42;1:235–40.

39 Moeller, SM *et al.* 2000. The potential role of dietary xanthophylls in cataract and age-related macular degeneration. *J Am Coll Nutr* 19:(5 Suppl):522S–527S.

40 Chasan-Taber, L *et al.* 1999. A prospective study of carotenoid and vitamin A intakes and risk of cataract extraction in US women. *Am J Clin Nutr* 70;4:509–16.

41 Paolisso, G *et al.* 1994. Plasma vitamin C affects glucose homeostasis in healthy subjects and in non-insulin-dependent diabetics. *Am J Physiol* 266:E261–8.

42 Paolisso, G, *et al.* 1995. Metabolic benefits deriving from chronic vitamin C supplementation in aged non-insulin dependent diabetics. *J Am Coil Nutr* 14:387–92.

43 Hutchinson, ML, Lee, WYL, Chen, MS *et al.* 1983. Effects of glucose and select pharmacologic agents on leukocyte ascorbic acid levels. *Fed Proc.* 42:930.

44 Secher, K. 1942. The bearing of the ascorbic acid content of the blood on the course of the blood sugar curve. *Acta Med Scand.* 60:255–65.

45 Davie, SJ, Gould, BJ, Yudkin, JS. 1992. Effect of vitamin C on glycosylation in diabetes. *Diabetes* 41:167–73.

46 Wang, H *et al.* 1995. Experimental and clinical studies on the reduction of erythrocyte sorbitol-glucose ratios by ascorbic acid in diabetes mellitus. *Diabetes Res Clin Pract* 28:1–8.

47 Vinson, JA, Staretz, ME, Bose, P *et al.* 1989. In vitro and in vivo reduction of erythrocyte sorbitol by ascorbic acid. *Diabetes.* 38:1036–41.

48 Cunningham, JJ *et al.* 1994. Vitamin C: An aldose reductase inhibitor that normalizes erythrocyte sorbitol in insulin-dependent diabetes mellitus. *J Am Coil Nutr* 13:344–50.

49 Ginter, E *et al.* 1978. Hypocholesterolemic effect of ascorbic acid in maturity-onset diabetes mellitus. *Int J Vitam Nutr Res* 48:368–73.

50 Paolisso, G, Balbi, V, Volpe, C *et al.* 1995. Metabolic benefits deriving from chronic vitamin C supplementation in aged non

insulin dependent diabetics. *J Am Coll Nutr* 14:387–92.

51 Eriksson, J and Kohvakka, A. 1995. Magnesium and ascorbic acid supplementation in diabetes mellitus. *Ann Nutr Metab* 39:217–23.

52 Simon, JA, Hudes, ES, Browner, WS. 1998. Serum ascorbic acid and cardiovascular disease prevalence in US adults. *Epidemiology* 9;3:316–21.

53 Jacob, RA. 1998. Vitamin C nutriture and risk of atherosclerotic heart disease. *Nutr Rev* 56;11:334–7.

54 Riemersma, RA *et al.* 1991. Risk of angina pectoris and plasma concentrations of vitamins A, C and E and carotene. *Lancet.* 337:1–5.

55 Nyyssonen, K. 1997 Vitamin C deficiency and risk of myocardial infarction: prospective population study of men from eastern Finland. *BMJ.* 314:634–638.

56 Khaw, K-T *et al.* 2001. Relation between plasma ascorbic acid and mortality in men and women in EPIC-Norfolk prospective population study. *Lancet* 357:657–63.

57 Gale, CR *et al.* Vitamin C and risk from stroke and coronary heart disease in cohort of elderly people. *BMJ* 1995; 310:1563–1566.

58 Timimi FK *et al.* 1998. Vitamin C improves endothelium-dependent vasodilation in patients with insulin-dependent diabetes mellitus. *Journal of the American College of Cardiology.* 31;3:552–57.

59 Ting, HH *et al.* 1996 Vitamin C improves endothelium-dependent vasodilation in patients with non-insulin-dependent diabetes mellitus. *J Clin Invest* 97:22–8.

60 Leske, MC *et al.* 1991. The lens opacities case-control study: Risk factors for cataract. *Arch Ophthalmol* 109;2:244–51.

61 Robertson, J McD, Donner, AP, Trevithick, JR. 1991. A possible role for vitamins C and E in cataract prevention. *Am J Clin Nutr.* 53:346S-51S.

62 Hankinson, S *et al.* 1992. Nutrient intake and cataract extraction in women: a prospective study. *BMJ* 305:335–9.

63 Jacques, PF *et al.* 1997. Long-term vitamin C supplement use and prevalence of early age-related lens opacities. *Am J Clin Nutr* 66 (4) p911–6.

64 Carr, AC, Frei, B. 1999. Toward a new recommended dietary allowance for vitamin C based on antioxidant and health effects in humans. *Am J Clin Nutr* 69:6:1086–1107.

65 Levine, M *et al.* 1999. Criteria and recommendations for vitamin C intake. *JAMA.* 281(15):1415–23.

66 Will, JC, Byers, T. 1996. Does diabetes mellitus increase the requirement for vitamin C? *Nutr Rev* 54;7:193–202.

67 Sinclair, AJ *et al.* 1994. Low plasma ascorbate levels in patients with type II diabetes mellitus consuming adequate dietary vitamin C. *Diabet Med* 11:893–8.

68 McCarty, MF. 1999. Can correction of sub-optimal coenzyme Q status improve beta-cell function in type II diabetics? *Med Hypotheses* 52;5:397–400.

69 Serebruany, VL *et al.* 1997. *J Cardiovasc Pharmacol* 29(1) 16–22.

70 Watts, GF *et al.* 2002. Coenzyme Q10 improves endothelial dysfunction of the brachial artery in Type II diabetes mellitus. *Diabetologia.* 45;3:420–6.

71 Fujioka, T *et al.* 1983. Clinical study of cardiac arrhythmias using a 24-hour continuous electrocardiographic recorder (5th report) – antiarrhythmic action of coenzyme Q10 in diabetics. *Tohoku J Exp Med.* 141 Suppl:453–63.

72 Munkholm, H *et al.* 1999. Coenzyme Q10 treatment in serious heart failure. *Biofactors* 9(2–4) 285–9.

73 Morisco, C *et al.* 1993. Effect of coenzyme Q10 therapy in patients with congestive heart failure: a long-term multicenter randomized study. *Clin Investig* 71 (8 Suppl) S134–6.

74 Langsjoen, H *et al.* 1994. Usefulness of coenzyme Q10 in clinical cardiology: a long-term study. *Mol Aspects Med* 15 Suppl S165–75.

75 Digiesi, V *et al.* 1990. Effect of coenzyme Q10 on essential arterial hypertension. *Curr Ther Res.* 47:841–845.

76 Langsjoen, P *et al.* 1994. Treatment of essential hypertension with coenzyme Q10. *Mol Aspects Med.* 15 Suppl S265–72.

77 Hodgson, JM *et al.* 2002. Coenzyme Q10 improves blood pressure and glycaemic control: a controlled trial in subjects with type 2 diabetes. *Eur J Clin Nutr.* 56;11:1137–42.

78 Miyake, Y. 1999. Effect of treatment with 3-hydroxy-3-methyl-glutaryl coenzyme A reductase inhibitors on serum coenzyme Q10 in diabetic patients. *Arzneimittelforschung* 49;4:324–9.

79 Fuller, CJ, Chandalia, M *et al.* 1996. RRR-alpha-tocopheryl acetate supplementation at pharmacologic doses decreases low-density-liproprotein oxidative susceptibility but not protein glycation in patients with diabetes mellitus. *Am J Clin Nutr*, 63: 753–9.

80 Jain, SK, McVie, R *et al.* 1996. The effect of modest vitamin E supplementation on lipid peroxidation products and other cardiovascular risk factors in diabetic patients. *Lipids* 315:

S87–90; and Jain SK, McVie R *et al.* Effect of modest vitamin E supplementation on blood glycated haemoglobin and triglyceride levels and red cellindices in type 1 diabetic patients. *J Am Coll Nutr.* 15;5:458–61.

81 Bierenbaum, ML *et al.* The effect of supplemental vitamin E on serum parameters in diabetics, post coronary and normal subjects. *Nutr Rep Internat* 31:1171–80, 1985.

82 Paolisso, G *et al.* Pharmacologic doses of vitamin E improve insulin action in healthy subjects and non-insulin dependent diabetic patients. *Am J Clin Nutr* 57:650–6, 1993.

83 Paolisso, G *et al.* Daily vitamin E supplements improve metabolic control but not insulin secretion in elderly type II diabetic patients. *Diabetes Care* 16:1433–7, 1993.

84 Paolisso G *et al.* 1993. Pharmacologic doses of vitamin E improve insulin action in healthy subjects and non-insulin dependent diabetic patients. *Am J Clin Nutr,* 1993; 57: 650–56.

85 Salonen, JT *et al.* 1995. Increased risk of non-insulin dependent diabetes mellitus at low plasma vitamin E concentrations: A four year follow up study in men. *BMJ.* 311;7013:1124–7.

86 Duntas, L *et al.* 1996. Administration of d-alphatocopherol in patients with insulin-dependent diabetes mellitus. *Curt Ther Res* 57:682–90.

87 Eg Shoff, SM *et al.* 1993. Glycosylated haemoglobin concentrations and vitamin E, vitamin C, and beta-carotene intake in diabetic and nondiabetic older adults. *Am J Clin Nutr,* 58:412–16.

88 Ceriello, A, Giugliano, D, Quatraro, A *et al.* 1991. Vitamin E reduction of protein glycosylation in diabetes. *Diabetes Care* 14:68–72.

89 Duntas, L *et al.* 1996. Administration of d-alpha-tocopherol in patients with insulin-dependent diabetes mellitus. *Curr Ther Res* 57:682–90.

90 Reaven, PD *et al.*: Effect of vitamin E on susceptibility of low-density lipoprotein and low-density lipoprotein subfractions to oxidation and on protein glycation in NIDDM. *Diabetes Care* 18:807, 1995.

91 Paolisso, G *et al.* 1993. Daily vitamin E supplements improve metabolic control but not insulin secretion in elderly type 2 diabetic patients. *Diabetes Care* 16:1433–7.

92 Colette, C *et al.* 1988. Platelet function in type I diabetes: effects of supplementation with large doses of vitamin E. *Am J Clin Nutr* 47:256–61.

93 Gisnger, C, Jeremy, J, Speiser, P *et al.* 1988. Effect of vitamin E supplementation on platelet thromboxane A2 production in type I diabetic patients: Double-blind crossover trial. *Diabetes* 37:1260–4.

94 Gey, KF *et al.* 1989. Plasma vitamin E and A inversely correlated to mortality from ischaemic heart disease in cross-cultural epidemiology. *Ann NY Acad Sci* 570:268–282.

95 Stampfer, MJ *et al.* 1993. Vitamin E consumption and the risk of coronary heart disease in women. *N Engl J Med* 328:1444–1449.

96 Rimm, EB *et al.* 1993. Vitamin E consumption and the risk of coronary heart disease in men. *N Eng J Med* 328:1450–1456.

97 Stephens, NG *et al.* 1996. Randomised controlled trial of vitamin E in patients with coronary disease: Cambridge Heart Antioxidant Study (CHAOS). *Lancet* 347:781–785.

98 Schmidt, R *et al.* 1998. Plasma antioxidants and cognitive performance in middle aged and older adults: results of the Austrian stroke prevention study. *J Am Geriat Soc* 46:1407–1410.

99 Tavani, A *et al.* 1996. Food and nutrient intake and risk of cataract. *Ann Epidemiol.* 6;1:41–6.

100 Leske, MC *et al.* 1991. The lens opacities case-control study: Risk factors for cataract. *Arch Ophthalmol* 109;2:244–51.

101 Rizvi, SI, Zaid, MA. 2001. Insulin-like effect of (-)epicatechin on erythrocyte membrane acetylcholinesterase activity in type 2 diabetes mellitus. *Clin Exp Pharmacol Physiol* 28;9:776–8.

102 Hosoda, K *et al.* 2003. Antihyperglycemic effect of oolong tea in type 2 diabetes. *Diabetes Care.* 26;6:1714–8.

103 Gomes, A *et al.* 1995. Anti-hyperglycemic effect of black tea (*Camellia sinensis*) in rat. *J Ethnopharmacol.* 45;3:223–6.

104 Hakim, IA *et al.* 2003. Tea consumption and the prevalence of coronary heart disease in Saudi adults: Results from a Saudi national study. *Prev Med.* 36;1:64–70.

105 Sesso, HD *et al.* 1999. Coffee and tea intake and the risk of myocardial infarction. *Am J Epidemiol.* 149;2:162–7.

106 Sasazuki, S *et al.* 2000. Relation between green tea consumption and the severity of coronary atherosclerosis among Japanese men and women. *Ann Epidemiol.* 10;6:401–8.

107 Ryu, E. 1980. Prophylactic effect of tea on pathogenic micro-organism infection to human and animals. (Growth inhibitive and bacteriocidal effect of tea on food poisoning and other path-ogenic enterobacterium in vitro.) *Int J Zoonoses.* 7;2:164–70.

108 Fassina, G *et al.* 2002. Polyphenolic antioxidant (-)-epigallocate-

chin-3-gallate from green tea as a candidate anti-HIV agent. *AIDS* 16;6:939–41.

109 Weber, JM *et al.* 2003. Inhibition of adenovirus infection and adenain by green tea catechins. *Antiviral Res.* 58;2:167–73.

110 Chida M *et al.* 1999. In vitro testing of antioxidants and biochemical end-points in bovine retinal tissue. *Ophthal Res* 31;6:407–415.

111 Liu, X *et al.* 2004. French maritime pine bark extract Pycnogenol dose-dependently lowers glucose in Type 2 diabetic patients. *Diabetes Care* 27;3:839.

112 Liu, X *et al.* 2004. Antidiabetic effect of French maritime pine bark extract Pycnogenol in patients with Type 2 diabetes. *Life Sci* 8;75;21:2505–13

113 Schonlau, F, Rohdewald, P. 2001. Pycnogenol for diabetic retinopathy: A review. *Int Ophthalmol.* 24;3:161–71.

114 Spadea, L, Balestrazzi, E. 2001. Treatment of vascular retinopathies with Pycnogenol. *Phytother Res* May;15(3):219–23.

115 Putter, M *et al.* 1999. Inhibition of smoking-induced platelet aggregation by aspirin and Pycnogenol. *Thromb Res* Aug 15 95(4):155–61.

116 Kljai, K, Runje, R. 2001. Selenium and glycogen levels in diabetic patients. *Biol Trace Elem Res* 83(3):223–9.

117 Ekmekcioglu, C *et al.* 2001. Concentrations of seven trace elements in different hematological matrices in patients with type 2 diabetes as compared to healthy controls. *Biol Trace Elem Res* 79(3):205–19.

118 Ruiz, C *et al.* 1998. Selenium, zinc and copper in plasma of patients with type 1 diabetes mellitus in different metabolic control states. *J Trace Elem Med Biol* 12;2:91–5.

119 Osterode, W *et al.* 1996. Nutritional antioxidants, red cell membrane fluidity and blood viscosity in type 1 (insulin dependent) diabetes mellitus. *Diabet Med* 13(12):1044–50.

120 Agren, MS *et al.* 1986. Selenium, zinc, iron and copper levels in serum of patients with arterial and venous leg ulcers. *Acta Derm Venereol* 66;3:237–40.

121 Stapleton, SR. 2000. Selenium: an insulin-mimetic. *Cell Mol Life Sci* Dec;57(13–14):1874–9.

122 Huttunene, JK. 1997. Selenium and cardiovascular diseases – an update. *Biomed Environ Sci* 10:2–3, 220–6.

123 Ricetti MM *et al.* 1999. Effects of sodium selenite on in vitro interactions between platelets and endothelial cells. *Int J Clin Lab Res* 29(2) 80–4.

124 Uden, S *et al.* 1990. Antioxidant therapy for recurrent pancreatitis: placebo-controlled trial. *Aliment Pharmacol Terap* 4;4:357–371, and see Bowrey, DJ *et al.* 1999 Selenium deficiency and chronic pancreatitis:disease mechanism and potential for therapy. *HPB Surg* 11(4) 207–15 and Morris-Stiff, GJ. 1999. The antioxidant profiles of patients with recurrent acute and chronic pancreatitis. *Am J Gastroenterol* 94(8) 2135–40.

125 Combs, GF *et al.* 1997. Reduction of cancer mortality and incidence by selenium supplementation. *Med Klin* 92 (Suppl 3 42–5).

126 Clark, LC *et al.* 1996. *JAMA* 276 (24) 1957–1963, and Clark, LC *et al.* 1998. Decreased evidence of prostate cancer with selenium supplementation: results of a double-blind cancer prevention trial. *Br J Urol* 81(5) 730–4.

127 Yoshizawa, K *et al.* 1998. Study of prediagnostic selenium level in toenails and the risk of advanced prostate cancer. *J Natl Cancer Inst.* 90 (16) 1219–24.

128 Rayman, M. 1997. Dietary selenium: time to act. *BMJ* 314:387–388.

CHAPTER 9

129 Verhoef, P *et al.* 1997. Plasma total homocysteine, B vitamins and risk of coronary atherosclerosis. *Arterioscler Thromb Vasc Biol* 17:989–95.

130 Refsum, H *et al.* 1998. Homocysteine and cardiovascular disease. *Ann Rev Med* 49:31–62.

131 Evers, S *et al.* 1997. Features, symptoms and neurophysiological findings in stroke associated with hyperhomocysteinemia. *Arch Neurol* 54:1276–82.

132 Ueland, PM *et al.* 2000. The controversy over homocysteine and cardiovascular risk. *Am J Clin Nutr* 72:324–32.

133 Boushey, CJ *et al.* 1995. A quantitative assessment of plasma homocysteine as a risk factor for vascular disease. Probable benefits of increasing folic acid intakes. *JAMA* 274:1049–57.

134 Graham, IM *et al.* 1997. Plasma homocysteine as a risk factor for vascular disease: The European Concerted Action Project. *JAMA* 277:1775–81.

135 Voutilainen, S *et al.* 1999. Enhanced in vivo lipid peroxidation at elevated plasma total homocysteine levels. *Arterioscler Thromb Vasc Biol* 19:1263–6.

136 Malinow, MR *et al.* 1999. Homocysteine, diet and cardiovascular disease: A statement for healthcare professionals from the

Nutrition Committee, American Heart Association. *Circulation* 99:178–82.

137 Pavia, C *et al.* 2000. Total homocysteine in patients with type 1 diabetes. *Diabetes Care* 23;1:84–7.

138 Meigs, JB *et al.* 2001. Fasting plasma homocysteine levels in the insulin resistance syndrome: The Framingham offspring study. *Diabetes Care* 24;8:1403–10.

139 Cenerelli, S *et al.* 2002. Helicobacter pylori masks differences in homocysteine plasma levels between controls and type 2 diabetic patients. *Eur J Clin Invest.* 32;3:158–62.

140 Emoto, M *et al.* 2001. Impact of insulin resistance and nephropathy on homocysteine in type 2 diabetes. *Diabetes Care* 24:533–538.

141 Hultberg, B *et al.* 1997. Poor metabolic control, early age at onset, and marginal folate deficiency are associated with increasing levels of plasma homocysteine in insulin-dependent diabetes mellitus: A five-year follow-up study. *Scand J Clin Lab Invest.* 57;7:595–600.

142 Baliga, BS *et al.* 2000. Hyperhomocysteinemia in type 2 diabetes mellitus: Cardiovascular risk factors and effect of treatment with folic acid and pyridoxine. *Endocr Pract* 6;6:435–41.

143 Ciccarone, E *et al.* 2003. Homocysteine levels are associated with the severity of peripheral arterial disease in Type 2 diabetic patients. *J Thromb Haemost.* 1;12:2540–7.

144 Merchant, AT *et al.* 2003. The use of B vitamin supplements and peripheral arterial disease risk in men are inversely related. *J Nutr.* 133;9:2863–7.

145 Ambrosch, A *et al.* 2001. Relation between homocysteinaemia and diabetic neuropathy in patients with Type 2 diabetes mellitus. *Diabet Med.* 18;3:185–92.

146 Buysschaert, M *et al.* 2000. Hyperhomocysteinemia in type 2 diabetes: Relationship to macroangiopathy, nephropathy, and insulin resistance. *Diabetes Care* 23;12:1816–1822.

147 Ozmen, B. 2002. Association between homocysteinemia and renal function in patients with type 2 diabetes mellitus. *Ann Clin Lab Sci.* 32;3:279–86.

148 Looker, HC *et al.* 2003. Homocysteine as a risk factor for nephropathy and retinopathy in Type 2 diabetes. *Diabetologia.* 46;6:766–72.

149 Becker, A *et al.* 2003. Plasma homocysteine and S-adenosylme-thionine in erythrocytes as determinants of carotid intima-media thickness: Different effects in diabetic and non-diabetic

individuals. The Hoorn Study. *Atherosclerosis.* 169;2:323–30.

150 de Luis, DA *et al.* 2002. Total homocysteine and cognitive deterioration in people with type 2 diabetes. *Diabetes Res Clin Pract* 55;3:185–90.

151 Passaro, A. 2003. Effect of metabolic control on homocysteine levels in type 2 diabetic patients: A 3-year follow-up. J Intern Med. 254;3:264–71.

152 Robinson, K *et al.* 1998. Low circulating folate and vitamin B6 concentrations: risk factors for stroke, peripheral vascular disease and coronary artery disease: European COMAC Group. *Circulation* 97:437–43.

153 Selhub, J *et al.* Vitamin status and intake as primary determinants of homocysteinemia in an elderly population. *JAMA* 1993;270:2693–8.

154 Homocysteine Lowering Trialists Collaboration. 1998. Lowering blood homocysteine with folic acid based supplements: Meta-analysis of randomised trials. *BMJ* 316:894–8.

155 Rydlewicz, A *et al.* 2002. The effect of folic acid supplementation on plasma homocysteine in an elderly population. *QJM* 95:27–35.

156 de Luis, DA *et al.* 2003. Relation between total homocysteine levels and beer intake in patients with diabetes mellitus Type 2. *Ann Nutr Metab.* 47;3–4:119–23.

157 Wulffele MG. 2003. Effects of short-term treatment with metformin on serum concentrations of homocysteine, folate and vitamin B12 in type 2 diabetes mellitus: A randomized, placebo-controlled trial. *J Intern Med.* 254;5:455–63.

158 Valerio, G *et al.* 1999. Lipophilic thiamine treatment in long-standing insulin-dependent diabetes mellitus. *Acta Diabetol.* 36;1–2:73–6.

159 Avena, R. 2000. Thiamine (Vitamin B1) protects against glucose- and insulin-mediated proliferation of human infragenicular arterial smooth muscle cells. *Ann Vasc Surg.* 14;1:37–43.

160 Obrenovich, ME, Monnier, VM. 2003. Vitamin B1 blocks damage caused by hyperglycemia. *Sci Aging Knowledge Environ* 10:PE6.

161 Hammes, HP *et al.* 2003. Benfotiamine blocks three major pathways of hyperglycemic damage and prevents experimental diabetic retinopathy. *Nat Med.* 9;3:294–9.

162 Saito, N *et al.* 1987. Blood thiamine levels in outpatients with diabetes mellitus. *J Nutr Sci Vitaminol (Tokyo)* 33;6:421–30.

163 Havivi, E *et al.* 1991. Vitamins and trace metals status in non

insulin dependent diabetes mellitus. *Int J Vitam Nutr Res* 61;4:328–33.

164 Havivi, E *et al.* 1991. Vitamins and trace metals status in non insulin dependent diabetes mellitus. *Int J Vitam Nutr Res* 61;4:328–33.

165 Cole, HS *et al.* 1976. Riboflavin deficiency in children with diabetes mellitus. *Acta Diabetol Lat.*13;1–2:25–9.

166 Kodentsova, VM *et al.* 1994. Vitamin metabolism in children with insulin-dependent diabetes mellitus: Effect of length of illness, severity, and degree of disruption of substance metabolism. *Vopr Med Khim* 40;4:33–8.

167 Kodentsova, VM *et al.* 1993. Metabolism of riboflavin and B group vitamins functionally bound to it in insulin-dependent diabetes mellitus. *Vopr Med Khim* 39;5:33–6.

168 Malaisse, WJ. 1993. Is type 2 diabetes due to a deficiency of FAD-linked glycerophosphate dehydrogenase in pancreatic islets? *Acta Diabetol* 30(1):1–5.

169 Head, KA. 2001. Natural therapies for ocular disorders, part two: Cataracts and glaucoma. *Altern Med Rev* 6;2:141–66.

170 Leske, MC *et al.* 1991. The lens opacities case-control study: Risk factors for cataract. *Arch Ophthalmol* 109;2:244–51.

171 Malik, S, Kashyap, ML. 2003. Niacin, lipids, and heart disease. *Curr Cardiol Rep* 5;6:470–6.

172 Pan, J *et al.* 2002. Extended-release niacin treatment of the atherogenic lipid profile and lipoprotein(a) in diabetes. *Metabolism* 51;9:1120–7.

173 Grundy, SM *et al.* 2002. Efficacy, safety, and tolerability of once-daily niacin for the treatment of dyslipidemia associated with type 2 diabetes: Results of the assessment of diabetes control and evaluation of the efficacy of niaspan trial. *Arch Intern Med* 162;14:1568–76.

174 Desouza, C *et al.* 2002. Drugs affecting homocysteine metabolism: impact on cardiovascular risk. *Drugs* 62;4:605–16.

175 Kane, MP *et al.* 2001. Cholesterol and glycemic effects of Niaspan in patients with type 2 diabetes. *Pharmacotherapy* 21;12:1473–8.

176 Rimm, EB *et al.* 1998. Folate and vitamin B6 from diet and supplements in relation to risk of coronary heart disease among women. *JAMA* 279;5:359–64.

177 Wilmink, AB *et al.* 2004. Dietary folate and vitamin B6 are independent predictors of peripheral arterial occlusive disease. *J Vasc Surg* 39;3:513–6.

178 McCann, VJ, Davis, RE. 1978. Serum pyridoxal concentrations in patients with diabetic neuropathy. *Aust N Z J Med* 8;3:259–61.

179 McCann, VJ, Davis, RE. 1978. Carpal tunnel syndrome, diabetes and pyridoxal. *Aust N Z J Med* 8;6:638–40.

180 Ellis, JM *et al.* 1991. A deficiency of vitamin B6 is a plausible molecular basis of the retinopathy of patients with diabetes mellitus. *Biochem Biophys Res Commun.* 179;1:615–9.

181 Havivi, E *et al.* 1991. Vitamins and trace metals status in non insulin dependent diabetes mellitus. *Int J Vitam Nutr Res* 61;4:328–33.

182 Davis, RE *et al.* 1976. Serum pyridoxal and folate concentrations in diabetics. *Pathology* 8:151–56.

183 Wilson, RG, Davis, RE. 1977. Serum pyridoxal concentrations in patients with diabetes mellitus. *Pathology* 9:95–98.

184 Rao, RH *et al.* 1980. Failure of pyridoxine to improve glucose tolerance in diabetics. *J Clin Endocrinol Metab* 50;1:198–200.

185 Solomon, LR, Cohen, K. 1989. Erythrocyte O2 transport and metabolism and effects of vitamin B6 therapy in type II diabetes mellitus. *Diabetes* 38:881–86.

186 Bauman, WA *et al.* 2000. Increased intake of calcium reverses vitamin B12 malabsorption induced by metformin. *Diabetes Care.* 23;9:1227–31.

187 Perros, P *et al.* 2000. Prevalence of pernicious anaemia in patients with Type 1 diabetes mellitus and autoimmune thyroid disease. *Diabet Med.* 17;10:749–51.

188 Looker, HC *et al.* 2003. Homocysteine as a risk factor for nephropathy and retinopathy in Type 2 diabetes. *Diabetologia.* 46;6:766–72.

189 Kornerup, T, Strom, L. 1958. Vitamin B12 and retinopathy in juvenile diabetics. *Acta Paediatr* 47:646–51.

190 Cameron, AJ, Ahern, GJ. 1958. Diabetic retinopathy and cyanocobalamin (vitamin B12): A preliminary report. *Br J Ophthalmal* 42:686–93.

191 Rimm, EB *et al.* 1998. Folate and vitamin B6 from diet and supplements in relation to risk of coronary heart disease among women. *JAMA.* 279;5:359–64.

192 Ajabnoor, MA *et al.* 2003. Homocysteine level and other biochemical parameters in cardiovascular disease patients with diabetes mellitus. *Med Sci Monit.* 9;12:CR523–7.

193 Wilmink, AB *et al.* 2004. Dietary folate and vitamin B6 are independent predictors of peripheral arterial occlusive disease. *J Vasc Surg.* 39;3:513–6.

194 Molgaard, J *et al.* 1992. Hyperhomocyst(e)inaemia: an independent risk factor for intermittent claudication. *J Intern Med.* 231;3:273–9.

195 Fiorina, P *et al.* 1998. Plasma homocysteine and folate are related to arterial blood pressure in type 2 diabetes mellitus. *Am J Hypertens.* 11;9:1100–7.

196 Woo, KS *et al.* 1999. Folic acid improves arterial endothelial function in adults with hyperhomocystinemia. *J Am Coll Cardiol.* 34;7:2002–6.

197 He, K *et al.* 2004. Folate, vitamin B6, and B12 intakes in relation to risk of stroke among men. *Stroke.* 35;1:169–74.

198 Tavani, A *et al.* 1996. Food and nutrient intake and risk of cataract. *Ann Epidemiol.* 6;1:41–6.

199 Havivi, E *et al.* 1991. Vitamins and trace metals status in non insulin dependent diabetes mellitus. *Int J Vitam Nutr Res.* 61;4:328–33.

200 Furukawa, Y. 1999. Enhancement of glucose-induced insulin secretion and modification of glucose metabolism by biotin. *Nippon Rinsho.* 57;10:2261–9.

201 Koutsikos, D *et al.* 1996. Oral glucose tolerance test after high-dose IV biotin administration in normoglucemic hemodialysis patients. *Ren Fail.* 18;1:131–7.

202 Coggeshall, JC *et al.* 1985. Biotin status and plasma glucose in diabetics. *Ann NY Acad Sci* 447:389–92.

203 Maebashi, M *et al.* 1993. Therapeutic evaluation of the effect of biotin on hyperglycemia in patients with non-insulin dependent diabetes mellitus. *J Clin Biochem Nutr.* 14:211–218.

204 Koutsikos, D *et al.* 1990. Biotin for diabetic peripheral neuropathy. *Biomed Pharmacother.* 44;10:511–514.

205 Strom, CM, Levine, EM. 1998. Chronic vaginal candidiasis responsive to biotin therapy in a carrier of biotinidase deficiency. *Obstet Gynecol.* 92;4 Pt 2:644–6.

CHAPTER 10

206 Davis, S *et al.* 1997. Age-related decreases in chromium levels in 51,665 hair, sweat, and serum samples from 40,872 patients: implications for the prevention of cardiovascular disease and type II diabetes mellitus. *Metabolism* 46:469–73.

207 Preuss, HG. 1997. Effects of glucose/insulin perturbations on aging and chronic disorders of aging: the evidence. *J Am Coll Nutr.* 16;5:397–403.

208 Ekmekcioglu, C *et al.* 2001. Concentrations of seven trace

elements in different hematological matrices in patients with type 2 diabetes as compared to healthy controls. *Biol Trace Elem Res.* 79(3):205–19.

209 Rukgauer, M, Zeyfang, A. 2002. Chromium determinations in blood cells: Clinical relevance demonstrated in patients with diabetes mellitus type 2. *Biol Trace Elem Res* 86;3:193–202.

210 Morris, BW *et al.* 1999. Chromium homeostasis in patients with type II (NIDDM) diabetes. *J Trace Elem Med Biol.* 13;1–2:57–61.

211 Anderson, RA *et al.* 2001. Potential antioxidant effects of zinc and chromium supplementation in people with type 2 diabetes mellitus. *J Am Coll Nutr* Jun;20(3):212–8.

212 Glinsmann, WH, Mertz, W. 1966. Effect of trivalent chromium on glucose tolerance. *Metabolism* 15:510–9.

213 Martinez, OB *et al.* 1985. Dietary chromium and effect of chromium supplementation on glucose tolerance of elderly Canadian women. *Nutr Res* 5:609–20.

214 Potter, JF *et al.* 1985. Glucose metabolism in glucose-intolerant older people during chromium supplementation. *Metabolism* 34:199–204.

215 Levine, RA *et al.* 1968. Effects of oral chromium supplementation on the glucose tolerance of elderly human subjects. *Metabolism* 17:114–25.

216 Jeejeebhoy, KN *et al.* 1977. Chromium deficiency, glucose intolerance, and neuropathy reversed by chromium supplementation in a patient receiving long-term total parenteral nutrition. *Am J Clin Nutr* 30:531–8.

217 Anderson, RA. 2000. Chromium in the prevention and control of diabetes. *Diabetes Metab* 26;1:22–7.

218 Davis, S, *et al.* 1997. Age-related decreases in chromium levels in 51,665 hair, sweat, and serum samples from 40,872 patients: implications for the prevention of cardiovascular disease and type II diabetes mellitus. *Metabolism* 46:469–73.

219 Anderson, RA *et al.* 1997. Elevated intakes of supplemental chromium improve glucose and insulin variables with type 2 diabetes. *Diabetes* 46:1786–91.

220 Fox, GN, Sabovic, Z. 1998. Chromium picolinate supplementation for diabetes mellitus. *J Fam Pract* 46:83–6.

221 Uusitupa, MIJ *et al.* 1983. Effect of inorganic chromium supplementation on glucose tolerance, insulin response, and serum lipids in noninsulin dependent diabetics. *Am J Clin Nutr* 38:404–410.

222 Simonoff, M. 1984. Chromium deficiency and cardiovascular

risk. *Cardiovasc Res.* 18;10:591–6.

223 Bahijiri, SM *et al.* 2000. The effects of inorganic chromium and brewer's yeast supplementation on glucose tolerance, serum lipids and drug dosage in individuals with type 2 diabetes. *Saudi Med J.* 21;9:831–7.

224 Abraham, AS *et al.* 1992. The effects of chromium supplementation on serum glucose and lipids in patients with and without non-insulin-dependent diabetes. *Metabolism.* 41;7:768–71.

225 Lee, NA, Reasner, CA. 1994. Beneficial effect of chromium supplementation on serum triglyceride levels in NIDDM. *Diabetes Care* 17:1449–52.

226 Kaats, GR *et al.* 1996. Effects of chromium picolinate supplementation on body composition: A randomized, double-masked, placebo-controlled study. *Curr Ther Res* 57:747–56.

227 Anderson, RA *et al.* 1992. Dietary chromium intake: freely chosen diets, institutional diets, and individual foods. *Biol Trace Elem Res* 32:117–21.

228 Urberg, M, Zemel, MB. 1987. Evidence for synergism between chromium and nicotinic acid in the control of glucose tolerance in elderly humans. *Metabolism* 36:896–9.

229 Anderson, RA *et al.* 1997. Lack of toxicity of chromium chloride and chromium picolinate. *J Am Coll Nutr* 16:273–9.

230 Zargar, AH *et al.* 1998. Copper, zinc, and magnesium levels in non-insulin dependent diabetes mellitus. *Postgrad Med J* 74;877:665–8.

231 Klevay, LM. 1982. An increase in glycosylated hemoglobin in rats deficient in copper. *Nutr Rep lnt* 26:329–34.

232 Wolf, WR *et al.* 1977. Daily intake of zinc and copper from self selected diets. *Fed Proc* 36:1175.

233 Ruiz, C *et al.* 1998. Selenium, zinc and copper in plasma of patients with type 1 diabetes mellitus in different metabolic control states. *J Trace Elem Med Biol* 12;2:91–5.

234 Klevay, LM *et al.* 1983. Diminished glucose tolerance in two men due to a diet low in copper. *Am J Clin Nutr* 37:717.

235 Klevay, LM *et al.* 1986. Decreased glucose tolerance in two men during experimental copper depletion. *Nutr Rep lnt* 33:371–82.

236 Klevay, LM. 1989. Ischemic heart disease as copper deficiency. *Adv Exp Med Biol* 258:197–208.

237 Klevay, LM. 1973. Hypercholesterolemia in rats produced by an increase in the ratio of zinc to copper ingested. *Am J Clin Nutr* 26:1060–1068.

238 Klevay, LM. 1998. Lack of a recommended dietary allowance for copper may be hazardous to your health. *J Am Coll Nutr* 17;4:322–6.

239 Klevay, LM. 1987. Dietary copper: a powerful determinant of cholesterolemia. *Med Hypotheses* 24;2:111–9.

240 Allen, KG, Klevay, LM. 1994. Copper: an antioxidant nutrient for cardiovascular health. *Curr Opin. Lipidol* 5: 22–28.

241 Ford, ES. 2000. Serum copper concentration and coronary heart disease among US adults. *Am J Epidemiol* 151;12:1182–8.

242 Salonen, JT *et al.* 1991. Serum copper and the risk of acute myocardial infarction: A prospective population study in men in eastern Finland. *Am J Epidemiol.* 134;3:268–76.

243 Klevay, LM. 1998. Lack of a recommended dietary allowance for copper may be hazardous to your health. *J Am Coll Nutr.* 17;4:322–6.

244 Lopez-Ridaura, R *et al.* 2004. Magnesium intake and risk of Type 2 diabetes in men and women. *Diabetes Care.* 27;1:134–140.

245 Song, Y *et al.* 2004. Dietary magnesium intake in relation to plasma insulin levels and risk of type 2 diabetes in women. *Diabetes Care.* 27;1:59–65.

246 Sjorgren, A *et al.* 1988. Oral administration of magnesium hydroxide to subjects with insulin dependent diabetes mellitus. *Magnesium* 121:16–20.

247 Barbagallo, M *et al.* 2003. Role of magnesium in insulin action, diabetes and cardio-metabolic syndrome X. *Mol Aspects Med* 24;1–3:39–52.

248 Kao, WH *et al.* 1999. Serum and dietary magnesium and the risk for type 2 diabetes mellitus: The Atherosclerosis Risk in Communities Study. *Arch Intern Med* 159;18:2151–9.

249 Guerrero-Romero, F, Rodriguez-Moran, M. 2002. Low serum magnesium levels and metabolic syndrome. *Acta Diabetol.* 39;4:209–13.

250 Rodriguez-Moran, M, Guerrero-Romero, F. 2003. Oral magnesium supplementation improves insulin sensitivity and metabolic control in type 2 diabetic subjects: A randomized double-blind controlled trial. *Diabetes Care.* 26;4:1147–52.

251 Ma, J *et al.* 1995. Associations of serum and dietary magnesium with cardiovascular disease, hypertension, diabetes, insulin, and carotid arterial wall thickness: The Atherosclerosis Risk in Communities Study. *J Clin Epidemiol* 48;7:927–40.

252 Chakraborti, S *et al.* 2002. Protective role of magnesium in cardiovascular diseases: A review. *Mol Cell Biochem*

238;1–2:163–79.

253 Corica, F *et al.* 1994. Effects of oral magnesium supplementation on plasma lipid concentrations in patients with non-insulin-dependent diabetes mellitus. *Magnes Res* Mar7;1:43–7.

254 Rodriguez-Moran, M, Guerrero-Romero, F. 2001. Low serum magnesium levels and foot ulcers in subjects with type 2 diabetes. *Arch Med Res* 32;4:300–3.

255 Morgan, KJ *et al.* 1985. Magnesium and calcium dietary intakes of the U.S. population. *J Am Coll Nutr* 4:195–206.

256 Walti, MK *et al.* 2003. Low plasma magnesium in type 2 diabetes. *Swiss Med Wkly* 133;19–20:289–92.

257 McNair, P *et al.* 1978. Hypomagnesemia, a risk factor in diabetic retinopathy. *Diabetes.* 27:1075–77.

258 Lima Mde L *et al.* 1998.The effect of magnesium supplementation in increasing doses on the control of type 2 diabetes. *Diabetes Care* 21;5:682–6.

259 Walti, MK *et al.* 2003. Measurement of magnesium absorption and retention in type 2 diabetic patients with the use of stable isotopes. *Am J Clin Nutr* 78;3:448–53.

260 Weder, AB. 1994. Sodium metabolism, hypertension, and diabetes. *Am J Med Sci* 307 Suppl 1:S53–9.

261 Singh, SK *et al.* 1999. Insulin resistance and urinary excretion of sodium in hypertensive patients with non-insulin dependent diabetes mellitus. *J Assoc Physicians India.* 47;7:709–11.

262 Nosadini, R *et al.* 1993. Role of hyperglycemia and insulin resistance in determining sodium retention in non-insulin-dependent diabetes. *Kidney Int* 44;1:139–46.

263 Gans, RO *et al.* 1992. Acute hyperinsulinemia induces sodium retention and a blood pressure decline in diabetes mellitus. *Hypertension* 20;2:199–209.

264 Quinones-Galvan, A, Ferranini, E 1997. Renal effects of insulin in man. *J Nephrol* 10;4:188–191.

265 Ames, RP. 2001. The effect of sodium supplementation on glucose tolerance and insulin concentrations in patients with hypertension and diabetes mellitus. *Am J Hypertens.* 14;7 Pt 1:653–9.

266 Petrie, JR. 1998. Dietary sodium restriction impairs insulin sensitivity in noninsulin-dependent diabetes mellitus. *J Clin Endocrinol Metab* 83;5:1552–7.

267 Lambert, J *et al.* 1997. Sodium, blood pressure, and arterial distensibility in insulin-dependent diabetes mellitus. *Hypertension* Nov;30(5):1162–8.

268 He FJ, MacGregor GA. 2002. Effect of modest salt reduction on blood pressure: a meta-analysis of randomized trials. Implications for public health. *J Human Hypertens* 16;11:761–70.

269 Elliott, P *et al.* 1996. Intersalt revisited: Further analyses of 24 hour sodium excretion and blood pressure within and across populations. Intersalt Cooperative Research Group. *BMJ* 312;7041:1249–53.

270 Stamler, J. 1997. The INTERSALT Study: Background, methods, findings, and implications. *Am J Clin Nutr* 65;2 Suppl:626S–642S.

271 Law, M. 2000. Salt, blood pressure and cardiovascular diseases. *J Cardiovasc Risk* 7;1:5–8.

272 Siani, A *et al.* 1991. Increasing the dietary potassium intake reduces the need for antihypertensive medication. *Ann Intern Med* 115;10:753–9.

273 Scientific Advisory Committee on Nutrition, Salt and Health. 2003. SACB/SaltSub/03/02:1–34.

274 Schmieder, RE, Messerli, FH. 2000. Hypertension and the heart. *J Human Hypertens* 14:597–604.

275 Safar, ME *et al.* 2000. Pressure-independent contribution of sodium to large artery structure and function in hypertension. *Cardiovasc Re* 46:269–276.

276 Simon, G *et al.* 2003. Development of structural vascular changes in salt-fed rats. *Am J Hypertens.* 16;6:488–93.

277 de Wardener, HE. 1990. The primary role of the kidney and salt intake in the aetiology of essential hypertension: Part 1. *Clin Sci* 79:193–200; Part 2: 289–297.

278 Lifton, RP, Geller, DS. 2001. Molecular mechanisms of human hypertension. *Cell* 104;545–556.

279 Law, M. 2000. Salt, blood pressure and cardiovascular diseases. *J Cardiovasc Risk* 7;1:5–8.

280 Heyliger, CE *et al.* 1985. Effect of vanadate on elevated blood glucose and depressed cardiac performance of diabetic rats. *Science* 1985; 227:1474–77.

281 Domingo, JL *et al.* 1994. Relationship between reduction in food intake and amelioration of hyperglycemia by oral vanadate in STZ-induced diabetic rats. *Diabetes* 4:1267.

282 Boden, G *et al.* 1996. Effects of vanadyl sulfate on carbohydrate and lipid metabolism in patients with non-insulin-dependent diabetes mellitus. *Metabolism* 45:1130–35.

283 Furnsinn, C *et al.* 1995. Improved glucose tolerance by acute vanadate but not by selenate exposure in genetically obese rats

(fa/fa). *Intl J of Obesity and Related Metab Disorders* 19;7:458–63.

284 Halberstam, M *et al.* 1996. Oral vanadyl sulfate improves insulin sensitivity in NIDDM but not in obese nondiabetic subjects. *Diabetes* 45:659–66.

285 Sakurai, H. 2002. A new concept: the use of vanadium complexes in the treatment of diabetes mellitus. *Chem Rec* 2;4:237–48.

286 Ekmekcioglu, C *et al.* 2001. Concentrations of seven trace elements in different hematological matrices in patients with type 2 diabetes as compared to healthy controls. *Biol Trace Elem Res* 79(3):205–19.

287 Chausmer, AB. 1998. Zinc, insulin and diabetes. *J Am Coll Nutr.* 17;2:109–15.

288 Goldberg, ED *et al.* 1992. Zinc content of pancreatic islets in diabetes. *Arkh Patol* 54;5:24–8.

289 Nakamura, T *et al.* 1991. Kinetics of zinc status in children with IDDM. *Diabetes Care* 14:553–7.

290 Pidduck, HG *et al.* 1970. Hyperzincuria of diabetes mellitus and possible genetic implications of this observation. *Diabetes* 19:240–7.

291 Singh, RB *et al.* 1998. Current zinc intake and risk of diabetes and coronary artery disease and factors associated with insulin resistance in rural and urban populations of North India. *J Am Coll Nutr* 17;6:564–70.

292 Rao, KVR *et al.* 1987. Effect of zinc sulfate therapy on control and lipids in type I diabetes. *JAPI* 35:52.

293 Anderson, RA *et al.* 2001. Potential antioxidant effects of zinc and chromium supplementation in people with type 2 diabetes mellitus. *J Am Coll Nutr* 20;3:212–8.

294 Chausmer, AB. 1998. Zinc, insulin and diabetes. *J Am Coll Nutr* 17;2:109–15.

CHAPTER 11

295 Ghannam, N *et al.* 1986. The antidiabetic activity of aloes: preliminary clinical and experimental observations. *Horm Res* 24;4:288–94.

296 Vogler, BK, Ernst, E. 1999. Aloe vera: a systematic review of its clinical effectiveness. *Br J Gen Pract* 49;447:823–8.

297 Abdullah, KM *et al.* 2003. Effects of Aloe vera on gap junctional intercellular communication and proliferation of human diabetic and nondiabetic skin fibroblasts. *J Altern Complement Med* 9;5:711–8.

298 Lietti, A, Forni, G. 1976. Studies on vaccinium myrtillus anthocyanosides. 1. Vasoprotective and anti-inflammatory activity. *Arzneim Forsch* 26:829–32.

299 Laplaud, PM *et al.* 1997. Antioxidant action of Vaccinium myrtillus extract on human low density lipoproteins in vitro: initial observations. *Fundam Clin Pharmacol* 11;1:35–40.

300 Perossini, M *et al.* 1987. Diabetic and hypertensive retinopathy therapy with *Vaccinium myrtillus* anthocyanosides. Double blind placebo-controlled clinical trial. *Ann Ottalmol Clin Ocul* 113:1173.

301 Scharrer, A, Ober, M. 1981. Anthocyanosides in the treatment of retinopathies. *Kiln Monatsbl* Augenheikld Beih 178:386–9.

302 Bravetti, G. 1989. Preventive medical treatment of senile cataract with vitamin E and anthocyanosides: Clinical evaluation. *Ann Ottalmol Clin Ocul* 115:109.

303 Khanna, P *et al.* 1981. Hypoglycemic activity of polypeptide-p from a plant source. *J Nat Prod* 44;6:648–55.

304 Basch, E *et al.* 2003. Bitter melon (*Momordica charantia*): A review of efficacy and safety. *Am J Health Syst Pharm* 60;4:356–9.

305 Leatherdale, BA *et al.* 1981. Improvement in glucose tolerance due to *Momordica charantia* (*karela*). *BMJ* 282;6279:1823–4.

306 Welihinda, J *et al.* 1986. Effect of *Momordica charantia* on the glucose tolerance in maturity onset diabetes. *J Ethnopharmacol* 17;3:277–82.

307 Srivastava, Y *et al.* 1993. Antidiabetic and adaptogenic properties of *Momordica charantia* extract: An experimental and clinical evaluation. *Phytother Res* 7:285–89.

308 Ahmad, N, *et al.* 1999. Effect of *Momordica charantia* (*Karolla*) extracts on fasting and postprandial serum glucose levels in NIDDM patients. *Bangladesh Med Res Counc Bull* 25;1:11–3.

309 Basch, E *et al.* 2003. Bitter melon (*Momordica charantia*): a review of efficacy and safety. *Am J Health Syst Pharm* 60;4:356–9.

310 Azad Khan, AK *et al.* 1979. *Coccinia indica* in the treatment of patients with diabetes mellitus. *Bangladesh Med Res Counc Bull* 5;2:60–6.

311 Kamble, SM *et al.* 1998. Influence of *Coccinia indica* on certain enzymes in glycolytic and lipolytic pathway in human diabetes. *Indian J Med Sci* 52;4:143–6.

312 Goel, V *et al.* 2004. Efficacy of a standardized Echinacea preparation (Echinilin) for treatment of the common cold: a randomized, double-blind, placebo controlled trial. *Clin Pharm Ther*

29;1:75–83.

313 Henneicke-von Zepelin, H *et al.* 1999. *Curr Med Res Opin* 15;3:214–27.

314 Sharma, RD *et al.* 1990. Effect of fenugreek seeds on blood glucose and serum lipids in type I diabetes. *Eur J Clin Nutr* 44;4:301–6.

315 Madar, Z *et al.* 1988. Glucose-lowering effect of fenugreek in non-insulin dependent diabetics. *Eur J Clin Nutr* 42;1:51–4.

316 Gupta, A *et al.* 2001. Effect of *Trigonella foenum-graecum* (fenugreek) seeds on glycaemic control and insulin resistance in type 2 diabetes mellitus: A double blind placebo controlled study. *J Assoc Physicians India* 49:1057–61.

317 Raghuram, TC *et al.* 1994. Effect of fenugreek seeds on intravenous glucose disposition in non-insulin dependent diabetic patients. *Phytotherapy Res* 8: 83–6.

318 Sharma, RD *et al.* 1990. Effect of fenugreek seeds on blood glucose and serum lipids in type I diabetes. *Eur J Clin Nutr* 44;4:301–6.

319 Bakhsh, R, Chughtai, MI. 1984. Influence of garlic on serum cholesterol, serum triglycerides, serum total lipids and serum glucose in human subjects. *Nahrung* 28;2:159–63.

320 Ackermann, RT *et al.* 2001. Garlic shows promise for improving some cardiovascular risk factors. *Arch Intern Med* 161;6:813–24.

321 Silagy, C, Neil, AW. 1994. A meta-analysis of the effect of garlic on blood pressure. *The Journal of Hypertension* 12:463–468.

322 Silagy, C, Neil, AW 1994. Garlic as a lipid lowering agent – a meta-analysis. *J R Coll Phys London* 28:39–45.

323 Mader, FH. 1990. Treatment of hyperlipidemia with garlic powder tablets. *Arzneim-Forsch Drug Res* 40:1111–1116.

324 Koscielny, J *et al.* 1999. The antiatherosclerotic effect of *Allium sativum. Atherosclerosis* 144:237–249.

325 Breithaupt-Grogler, K *et al.* 1997. Protective effect of chronic garlic intake on elastic properties of aorta in the elderly. *Circulation* 96:2649–2655.

326 Ou, CC *et al.* 2003. Protective action on human LDL against oxidation and glycation by four organosulfur compounds derived from garlic. *Lipids* 38;3:219–24.

327 Kudolo, GB. 2001. The effect of 3-month ingestion of Ginkgo biloba extract (EGb 761) on pancreatic beta-cell function in response to glucose loading in individuals with non-insulin-dependent diabetes mellitus. *J Clin Pharmacol.* 41;6:600–11.

328 Kudolo, GB *et al.* 2002. Effect of the ingestion of Ginkgo biloba

extract on platelet aggregation and urinary prostanoid excretion in healthy and Type 2 diabetic subjects. *Thromb Res.* 108;2–3:151–60.

329 Witte, S *et al.* 1992. Improvement of hemorheology with ginkgo biloba extract: Decreasing a cardiovascular risk factor. *Fortschr Med* 110;13:247–50.

330 Doly, M *et al.* 1992. Oxidative stress in diabetic retina. *EXS* 62:299–307.

331 Lanthony, P, Cosson, JP. 1988. The course of color vision in early diabetic retinopathy treated with Ginkgo biloba extract: A preliminary double-blind versus placebo study. *J Fr Ophtalmol* 11;10:671–4.

332 Lebuisson, DA *et al.* 1986. Treatment of senile macular degeneration with Ginkgo biloba extract: A preliminary double-blind drug vs. placebo study. *Presse Med* 15;31:1556–8.

333 Fies P, Dienel, A. 2002. Ginkgo extract in impaired vision – treatment with special extract EGb 761 of impaired vision due to dry senile macular degeneration. *Wien Med Wochenschr* 152;15–16:423–6.

334 Raabe, A *et al.* 1991. Therapeutic follow-up using automatic perimetry in chronic cerebroretinal ischemia in elderly patients: Prospective double-blind study with graduated dose ginkgo biloba treatment (EGb 761). *Klin Monatsbl Augenheilkd* 199;6:432–8.

335 Pittler, MH, Ernst, E. 2000 Ginkgo biloba extract for the treatment of intermittent claudication: a meta-analysis of randomized trials. *Am J Med.* 108;4:276–81.

336 Paick, JS, Lee, JH. 1996. An experimental study of the effect of ginkgo biloba extract on the human and rabbit corpus cavernosum tissue. *J Urol* 156;5:1876–80.

337 Sikora, R *et al.* 1989. Ginkgo biloba extract in the therapy of erectile dysfunction. *J Urol* 141:188A.

338 Sohn, M, Sikora, R 1991. Ginkgo biloba extract in the therapy of erectile dysfunction. *J Sex Ed Ther* 17;1:53–61.

339 Sohn, M, Sikora, R. 1991. Ginkgo biloba extract in the therapy of erectile dysfunction. *J Sec Educ Ther* 17:53–61.

340 Clostre, F. 1999. Ginkgo biloba extract (EGb 761): State of knowledge in the dawn of the year 2000. *Ann Pharm Fr* 57 Suppl 1:1S8–88.

341 Birks, J *et al.* 2002. Ginkgo biloba for cognitive impairment and dementia. *Cochrane Database Syst Rev* 4:CD003120.

342 Vuksan, V *et al.* 2001. Konjac-Mannan and American ginseng:

emerging alternative therapies for type 2 diabetes mellitus. *J Am Coll Nutr* 20;5 Suppl:370S–380S; discussion 381S–383S.

343 Sotanieme, EA *et al.* 1995. Ginseng therapy in non-insulin-dependent diabetic patients. *Diabetes Care* 18;10:1373–1375.

344 Vogler, BK *et al.* 1999. The efficacy of ginseng: A systematic review of randomised clinical trials. *Eur J Clin Pharmacol* 55;8:567–75.

345 Vuksan, V. 2000. American ginseng (*Panax quinquefolius L*) reduces postprandial glycemia in nondiabetic subjects and subjects with type 2 diabetes mellitus. *Arch Intern Med* 160;7:1009–13.

346 Vuksan, V *et al.* 2000. Similar postprandial glycemic reductions with escalation of dose and administration time of American ginseng in type 2 diabetes. *Diabetes Care* 23;9:1221–6.

347 Choi, HK *et al.* 1995. Clinical efficacy of Korean red ginseng for erectile dysfunction. *Int J Impot Res* 7;3:181–6.

348 Hong, B. 2002. A double-blind crossover study evaluating the efficacy of Korean red ginseng in patients with erectile dysfunction: A preliminary report. *J Urol* 168;5:2070–3.

349 Kiefer, D, Pantuso, T. 2003. Panax ginseng. *Am Fam Physician* Oct 15;68(8):1539–42.

350 Warren, RP *et al.* 1969. Inhibition of the sweet taste by *Gymnema sylvestre*. *Nature* 223:94–5.

351 Hellekant, G *et al.* 1985. Effects of gymnemic acid on the chorda tympani proper nerve responses to sweet, sour, salty and bitter taste stimuli in the chimpanzee. *Acta Physiol Scand* 124:399–408.

352 Ye, W, Liu, X *et al.* 2001. Antisweet saponins from *Gymnema sylvestre*. *J Nat Prod* 64;2:232–5.

353 Shanmugasundaram, ER *et al.* 1990. Use of *Gymnema sylvestre* leaf extract in the control of blood glucose in insulin-dependent diabetes mellitus. *J Ethnopharmacol* 30;3:281–94.

354 Baskaran, K *et al.* 1990. Antidiabetic effect of a leaf extract from *Gymnema sylvestre* in non-insulin-dependent diabetes mellitus patients. *J Ethnopharmacol* 30;3:295–300.

355 Satdive, RK *et al.* 2003. Antimicrobial activity of *Gymnema sylvestre* leaf extract. *Fitoterapia* 74;7–8:699–701.

356 Agrawal, P *et al.* 1996. Randomized placebo-controlled, single blind trial of holy basil leaves in patients with noninsulin-dependent diabetes mellitus. *Int J Clin Pharmacol Ther* 34;9:406–9.

357 Rai V *et al.* 1997. Effect of ocimum sanctum leaf powder on

blood lipoproteins, glycated protein and total amino acids in patients with non-insulin dependent diabetes mellitus. *J Nutr Environ Med*, 1997; 7: 113–8.

358 Budinsky, A *et al.* 2001. Regular ingestion of *Opuntia robusta* lowers oxidation injury. *Prostaglandins Leukot Essent Fatty Acids* 65;1:45–50.

359 Frati, AC *et al.* 1991. The effect of two sequential doses of *Opuntia streptacantha* upon glycemia. *Arch Invest Med* 22;3–4:333–6.

360 Frati-Munari, AC *et al.* 1989. Hypoglycemic action of *Opuntia streptacantha Lemaire*: Study using raw extracts. *Arch Invest Med* 20;4:321–5.

361 Wolfram, RM *et al.* 2002. Effect of prickly pear (*Opuntia robusta*) on glucose- and lipid-metabolism in non-diabetics with hyperlipidemia: A pilot study. *Wien Klin Wochenschr* 114;19–20:840–6.

CHAPTER 12

362 Jamal, GA. 1994. The use of GLA in the prevention and treatment of diabetic neuropathy. *Diabetic Med* 11:145–149.

363 Feskens, EJM *et al.* 1991. Inverse association between fish intake and risk of glucose intolerance in normoglycemic elderly men and women. *Diabetes Care* 14:935–41.

364 Stene, LC *et al.* 2003. Use of cod liver oil during the first year of life is associated with lower risk of childhood-onset type 1 diabetes: A large, population-based, case-control study. *Am J Clin Nutr* 78;6:1128–34.

365 Borkman, M *et al.* 1989. Effects of fish oil supplementation on glucose and lipid metabolism in NIDDM. *Diabetes* 38:1314–19.

366 Friday, KE *et al.* 1989. Elevated plasma glucose and lowered triglyceride levels from omega-3 fatty acid supplementation in Type II diabetes. *Diabetes Care* 12:276–81.

367 Vessby, B, Boberg, M. 1990. Dietary supplementation with n-3 fatty acids may impair glucose homeostasis in patients with non-insulin-dependent diabetes mellitus. *J Intern Med* 228:165–71.

368 Annuzzi, G *et al.* 1991. A controlled study on the effects of n-3 fatty acids on lipid and glucose metabolism in non-insulin-dependent diabetic patients. *Atherosclerosis* 87:65–73.

369 Morgan, WA *et al.* 1995. A comparison of fish oil or corn oil supplements in hyperlipidemic subjects with NIDDM. *Diabetes Care* 18:83–86.

370 Popp-Snijders, C *et al.* 1987. Dietary supplementation of omega-

3 polyunsaturated fatty acids improves insulin sensitivity in non-insulin-dependent diabetes. *Diabetes* Res 4:141–7.

371 Connor, WE *et al.* 1993. The hypotriglyceridemic effect of fish oil in adult-onset diabetes without adverse glucose control. *Ann N Y Acad Sci* 683:337–40.

372 Luostarinen, R *et al.* 1995. Vitamin E supplementation counteracts the fish oil-induced increase of blood glucose in humans. *Nutr Res* 15:953–68.

373 Dunstan, DW *et al.* 1997. The independent and combined effects of aerobic exercise and dietary fish intake on serum lipids and glycemic control in NIDDM: A randomized controlled study. *Diabetes Care* 20:913–21.

374 Farmer, A *et al.* 2001. Fish oil in people with type 2 diabetes mellitus. *Cochrane Database Syst Rev* 3:CD003205.

375 Montori, VM *et al.* 2000. Fish oil supplementation in type 2 diabetes: A quantitative systematic review. *Diabetes Care* 23;9:1407–15.

376 Friedberg, CE *et al.* 1998. Fish oil and glycemic control in diabetes: A meta-analysis. *Diabetes Care* 21;4:494–50.

377 Hiroyasu, I *et al.* 2001. Intake of fish and omega-3 fatty acids and risk of stroke in women. *JAMA* 285:304–312.

378 Valagussa, *et al.* 1999. Dietary supplementation with n-3 polyunsaturated fatty acids and vitamin E after myocardial infarction: Results of the GISSI-Prevention Trial. *Lancet* 354:447–455.

379 Christensen, JH *et al.* 2001. Marine n-3 fatty acids, wine intake and heart rate variability in patients referred for coronary angiography. *Circulation* 103:651–657.

380 Albert, CM *et al.* 2002. Blood levels of long-chain n-3 fatty acids and the risk of sudden death. *N Eng J Med* 346:1113–1118.

381 McVeigh, GE *et al.* 1994. Fish oil improves arterial compliance in non-insulin-dependent diabetes mellitus. *Arterioscler Thromb* 14;9:1425–9.

382 Miller, ME *et al.* 1987. Effect of fish oil concentrates on hemorheological and hemostatic aspects of diabetes mellitus: A preliminary study. *Thromb Res* 47;2:201–14.

383 Sheehan, JP *et al.* 1997. Effect of high fiber intake in fish oil-treated patients with non-insulin-dependent diabetes mellitus. *Am J Clin Nutr* 66;5:1183–7.

384 Laidlaw, M, Holub, BJ. 2003. Effects of supplementation with fish oil-derived n-3 fatty acids and g-linolenic acid on circulating plasma lipids and fatty acid profiles in women 1–3. *Am J Clin*

Nutr 77;1:37–42.

385 Uccella, R *et al.* 1989. Action of evening primrose oil on cardio-vascular risk factors in insulin-dependent diabetics. *Clin Ter* 129;5:381–8.

386 Morse, PF *et al.* 1989. Meta-analysis of placebo-controlled studies of the efficacy of Epogam in the treatment of atopic eczema: Relationship between plasma essential fatty acid changes and clinical response. *Br J Dermatol* 121:75–90.

387 Fiocchi A *et al.* 1994. The efficacy and safety of gamma-linolenic acid in the treatment of infantile atopic dermatitis. *J Int Med Res* 22;1:24–32.

388 Arisaka, M *et al.* 1991. Fatty acid and prostaglandin metabolism in children with diabetes mellitus II: The effect of evening primrose oil supplementation on serum fatty acid and plasma prostaglandin levels. *Prostaglandins Leukot Essent Fatty Acids* 43;3:197–201.

389 Jamal, GA. 1994. The use of gamma linolenic acid in the prevention and treatment of diabetic neuropathy. *Diabet Med* 11;2:145–49.

390 Jamal, GA, Carmichael, H. 1990. The effect of gamma-linolenic acid on human diabetic peripheral neuropathy: A double-blind placebo-controlled trial. *Diabet Med* 7;4:319–23.

391 Keen, H *et al.* 1993. Treatment of diabetic neuropathy with gamma-linolenic acid: The gamma-Linolenic Acid Multicenter Trial Group. *Diabetes Care* 16;1:8–15.

392 Holman, CP, Bell, AFJ. 1983. A trial of evening primrose oil in the treatment of chronic schizophrenia. *J Orthomol Psychiatr* 12:302–4.

393 Brown, JM, McIntosh, MK. 2003. Conjugated linoleic acid in humans: Regulation of adiposity and insulin sensitivity. *J Nutr* 133;10:3041–6.

394 Blankson, H *et al.* 2000. Conjugated linoleic acid reduces body fat mass in overweight and obese humans. *J Nutr* 130;12:2943–8.

395 Riserus, U *et al.* 2001. Conjugated linoleic acid (CLA) reduced abdominal adipose tissue in obese middle-aged men with signs of the metabolic syndrome: A randomised controlled trial. *Int J Obes Relat Metab Disord* 25;8:1129–35.

396 Noone, EJ *et al.* 2002. The effect of dietary supplementation using isomeric blends of conjugated linoleic acid on lipid metabolism in healthy human subjects. *Br J Nutr* 88;3:243–51.

APPENDIX 1

397 Manson, JE *et al.* 1991. Physical activity and incidence of noninsulin-dependent diabetes mellitus in women. *Lancet*
   338:774–778; Pan, XR *et al.* 1997. Effects of diet and exercise in
   preventing NIDDM in people with impaired glucose tolerance:
   The Da Qing IGT and Diabetes Study. *Diabetes Care*
   20;4:537–44.

398 Helmrich, SP *et al.* 1991. Physical activity and reduced occurrence of non-insulin-dependent diabetes mellitus. *N Engl J Med*
   325;3:147–52.

399 Lindstrom, J *et al.* 2003. Prevention of diabetes mellitus in
   subjects with impaired glucose tolerance in the Finnish diabetes
   prevention study: Results from a randomized clinical trial. *J Am
   Soc Nephrol* 14(7 Suppl 2):S108–13; Knowler, WC *et al.* 2002.
   Reduction in the incidence of type 2 diabetes with lifestyle intervention or metformin. *N Engl J Med* 346;6:393–403.

400 Tuomilehto, J *et al.* 2001. Prevention of type 2 diabetes mellitus
   by changes in lifestyle among subjects with impaired glucose
   tolerance. *N Engl J Med* 344:1343–50.

401 Boule, NG *et al.* 2001. Effects of exercise on glycemic control
   and body mass in type 2 diabetes mellitus: a meta-analysis of
   controlled clinical trials. *JAMA* 286:1218–27.

402 Borghouts, LB, Keizer, HA. 2000. Exercise and insulin sensitivity: A review. *Int J Sports Med* 21:1–12.

403 Ivy, JL. 1997. Role of exercise training in the prevention and
   treatment of insulin resistance and non-insulin-dependent
   diabetes mellitus. *Sports Med* 24;5:321–36.

404 Braun B *et al.* 1995. Effects of exercise intensity on insulin sensitivity in women with non-insulin-dependent diabetes mellitus. *J
   Appl Physiol.* 78;1:300–6.

405 Rogers MA *et al.* 1990. Effect of 10 days of physical inactivity
   on glucose tolerance in master athletes. *J Appl Physiol.* 68;5:
   1833–7.

406 King DS *et al.* 1995. Time course for exercise-induced alterations
   in insulin action and glucose tolerance in middle-aged people. *J
   Appl Physiol.* 78;1:17–22.

407 Ivy, JL. 1997. Role of exercise training in the prevention and
   treatment of insulin resistance and non-insulin-dependent
   diabetes mellitus. *Sports Med* 24;5:321–36.

408 Khayat, ZA *et al.* 2002. Exercise- and insulin-stimulated muscle
   glucose transport: distinct mechanisms of regulation. *Can J Appl*

Physiol 27;2:129–51; Dela, F *et al.* 1994. Effect of training on interaction between insulin and exercise in human muscle. *J Appl Physiol* 76;6:2386–93.

409 Goodyear, LJ, Kahn, BB. 1998. Exercise, glucose transport, and insulin sensitivity. *Annu Rev Med* 49:235–61.

410 Houmard, JA *et al.* 1991. Elevated skeletal muscle glucose transporter levels in exercise-trained middle-aged men. *Am J Physiol* 261(4 Pt 1):E437–43.

411 Price, TB *et al.* 1996. NMR studies of muscle glycogen synthesis in insulin-resistant offspring of parents with non-insulin-dependent diabetes mellitus immediately after glycogen-depleting exercise. *Proc Natl Acad Sci USA.* 93;11:5329–34.

412 Perseghin, G *et al.* 1996. Increased glucose transport-phosphorylation and muscle glycogen synthesis after exercise training in insulin-resistant subjects. *N Engl J Med* 335;18:1357–62.

413 Ivy, JL. 1997. Role of exercise training in the prevention and treatment of insulin resistance and non-insulin-dependent diabetes mellitus. *Sports Med* 24;5:321–36.

414 Helge, JW, Dela, F. 2003. Effect of training on muscle triacylglycerol and structural lipids: A relation to insulin sensitivity? *Diabetes* 52:1881–1887.

415 Lim, JG *et al.* 2004. Type 2 diabetes in Singapore: The role of exercise training for its prevention and management. *Singapore Med J* 45;2:62–8.

416 Borghouts, LB, Keizer, HA. 2000. Exercise and insulin sensitivity: A review. *Int J Sports Med* 21:1–12. van Baak, MA, Borghouts, LB. 2000. Relationships with physical activity. *Nutr Rev* 58(3 Pt 2):S16–8; Schneider, SH *et al.* 1984. Studies on the mechanism of improved glucose control during regular exercise in type 2 diabetes. *Diabetologia* 26:355–60.

APPENDIX 2

417 Scheen, AJ. Prevention of type 2 diabetes in obese patients: First results with orlistat in the XENDOS study. *Rev Med Liege* 2002 57;9:617–21.

APPENDIX 3

418 Gutierrez, M *et al.* 1998. Utility of a short term 25 per cent carbohydrate diet on improving glycemic control in Type 2 diabetes mellitus. *J Am Coll Nutr* 17(6):595–600.

419 Brehm, BJ *et al.* 2003 A randomised trial comparing a very low-

carbohydrate diet and a calorie-restricted low-fat diet on body weight and cardiovascular risk factors in healthy women. *J Clin Endocrinol Metab* 88;4:1617–1623.

420 Foster, GD *et al.* 2003. A randomised trial of a low-carbohydrate diet for obesity. *New Eng J Med* 348;21:2082–2090.

421 Samaha, FF *et al.* 2003. A low-carbohydrate as compared with a low-fat diet in severe obesity. *N Eng J Med* 348:21, 2074–81.

422 Stern, L *et al.* 2004. The effects of low-carbohydrate versus conventional weight loss diets in severely obese adults: One-year follow-up of a randomized trial. *Ann Intern Med* 140:778–785.

423 Westman, E *et al.* 2002. Effect of 6-month adherence to a very low-carbohydrate diet program. *Am J Med* 113:30–36.

424 Yancy, W *et al.* 2004. A low-carbohydrate, ketogenic diet versus a low-fat diet to treat obesity and hyperlipidemia: A randomised controlled trial. *Ann Intern Med* 140:769–777.

Bibliography

Atkins, Dr Robert C, *Atkins for Life*, Macmillan, 2003

Atkins, Dr Robert C, *The New Carbohydrate Counter*, Vermilion, 2003

Atkins, Dr Robert C, *Atkins Diabetes Revolution*, Thorsons, 2004

Atkins, Dr Robert C, *Atkins Made Easy: the first 2 weeks*, Thorsons, 2004

Brewer, Dr Sarah, *Encyclopedia of Vitamins, Minerals & Herbal Supplements*, Robinson, 2002

Brewer, Dr Sarah, *Eat to Beat High Blood Pressure*, Thorsons, 2003

Clarke, Dr Charles, *The New High Protein Diet*, Vermilion, 2002

Foster, Helen, *Easy GI Diet*, Hamlyn, 2004

Hillson, Dr Rowan, *Diabetes: A new guide*. Optima Positive Health Guide, 1992.

Holford, Patrick, and Braly, Dr James, *The H Factor*, Piatkus, 2003

McCully, Dr KM, *The Heart Revolution*, Harper Perennial, 1999

Sims, Dr Jeremy, *The Calorie, Carb & Fat Bible*, WLR/Penhaligon Page Ltd, www.weightlossresources.co.uk, 2002

Williams, Prof G and Pickup, Dr John C, *Handbook of Diabetes* (2nd Edn), Blackwell Science, 1999

Index

acarbose 46–7
ACE inhibitors 31, 59–60, 117
acetylcholine 33
adiponectin 54
age 12
age-related macular degeneration 110, 128, 211–12
agnus castus 115
albumin 11, 26, 126
alcohol consumption 49–50, 62, 87–8, 102, 157
allicin 209
aloe vera 35, 115, 196, 198–200
alpha-glucosidase inhibitors 46–7
alpha-linolenic acid (ALA) 77, 229
alpha-lipoic acid (ALA) 26, 27, 124–7, 238
Alzheimer's disease (AD) 22, 32–3, 213
American Diabetes Association (ADA) 15, 95
amino acids 73–5, 100
amputation 22, 35
amylin 10
anaemia
    iron-deficiency 110, 219
    pernicious 166, 168
androgens 40
angina 22, 29, 60, 103, 132
antacids 118
anthocyanosides 200–2
anthraquinones 199–200
anti-blood clotting agents 85
    see also aspirin; warfarin
    antioxidant 87, 120, 124, 136, 146–7
    essential fatty acids as 227–8, 230
    herbal 122, 196, 211
anti-epileptic drugs 28, 171
anti-inflammatories 85, 140, 225
anti-obesity drugs 66, 245–8
antibiotics 36, 38, 117–18, 173, 219
antidepressants 28, 119, 121, 217

antihypertensives 10–11, 25, 61, 63, 80–1, 91
    AB/CD rule 59–60
antioxidants 25–6, 29, 78, 111, 238
    definition 123
    dietary sources 63, 83–8
    herbal 201, 208–10
    supplementation 107–8, 123–49
apolipoproteins 162
apomorphine (Uprima) 37
apple-shaped figures (visceral fat) 12–13, 17, 19, 53, 92, 233, 241
artificial sweeteners 114, 218
aspartame 114
aspirin 27, 30, 66, 118, 121–2, 214
atherosclerosis 18, 22, 30, 79–80, 83, 85, 87, 144, 158, 182, 209, 212
Atkins diet (Atkins Nutritional Approach) 56, 64, 69, 98–104, 235, 249
autoimmune disorders 4, 8, 10

bed cradles 27
beer 157
benzodiazepines 28
beta blockers 10–11, 31, 59–60, 118
beta-cryptoxanthin 128
betacarotene 85, 123, 127–30
biguanides 45
bilberry 25, 34, 121, 196, 200–2, 238
biotin ix, 171–3
birth defects 110, 129, 166, 168, 170–1
birth weight, low 9
bitter melon 196, 202–4
blood clotting factors 18
    see also anti-blood clotting agents
blood pressure 58, 92, 103, 169
    see also high blood pressure
blood sugar (glucose)
    see also hypoglycaemic drugs, oral

balancing
  with antioxidants 124–5, 130–1,
      136, 138, 143, 145, 147
  with B vitamins 151, 171–2
  with diet 70–2, 98, 101
  with exercise 242–3
  with fibre 89
  with herbs 196, 198–9, 201–4,
      207–11, 214–16, 218–21
  importance of 21–3, 26–7, 30, 32,
      34, 36, 37, 40
  with minerals 175–8, 181, 184–5,
      191–3
diagnostic levels in diabetes 14–15
effect of fatty acids on 53–4, 224–8,
    233–4
elevated levels 1, 13, 19, 21–7, 36–9
and insulin resistance 4–5
and ketoacidosis 100–1
metabolism 1–3
monitoring 41, 44, 47–8, 93, 96,
    99–100, 105, 116, 127, 239
and premetabolic syndrome 17–18
and renal threshold 14
target levels 47
uptake 243
urinary secretion 6–7, 14
blood vessels 33–4
  see also atherosclerosis; vascular disease,
      peripheral
  damage to 18, 22, 24–6, 28–9, 60,
      131, 155, 190
  supplements for 128, 136–7, 140, 144,
      158, 185, 201
  treatment 34
body mass index (BMI) 54–5
bones 35, 110, 118
brain
  function 141, 155, 213
  haemorrhage 121–2
  inflammation 33
breakfasts 68, 69
breastfeeding 51, 79, 115, 199–200
bromelain 118
butter 82

caffeine 86, 87
calcium 110, 115, 118, 166, 174
calcium channel blockers 59–60
cancer 130
cancer-protective foods 85, 110, 124, 132,
    148, 168
captopril 117
carbamazepine 28

carbohydrates 70–3
  see also low-carbohydrate diets
  and coronary heart disease 103
  of low-fat diets 96–7
  simple/refined 4, 11–12, 17, 70
  slow-releasing/unrefined 68, 70
  traditional intake 67
cardiomyopathy 30
carotenoids 25, 85, 110, 123, 127–30
carpal tunnel syndrome 164–5
cataracts 24, 111, 128–9, 133–4, 141,
    151, 160, 170, 201
causes of diabetes 8–13
cell division 166, 168
cerebral retinal insufficiency, chronic 212
charantin 202
chest pain 29–30
children 44, 91, 128, 160, 165
chilli pepper 27
cholesterol absorption inhibitors 65
cholesterol levels
  herbs for 196, 201, 207–9, 218, 220–2
  high density lipoprotein (HDL) (good)
      and anti-obesity drugs 245
      and diet 79, 80, 82, 87
      essential fatty acids and 226, 227,
          230, 234
      low levels 18, 19, 22, 58, 63–4
      and low-carb diets 252–4
      micronutrients for 162, 178, 185
      and weight loss 92, 97, 98, 103
  low-density lipoprotein (LDL) (bad)
      and anti-obesity drugs 245
      effects of dietary fats on 76, 79–82,
          226–7, 229–30, 234
      high levels 22, 26, 30, 58, 60, 63–6
      and low carb-diets 252–4
      lowering with exercise 92
      lowering with supplements 131–2,
          139, 161–3, 178, 181–2,
          185
      and weight loss 92, 98, 103
  measuring levels 64
  very low density lipoprotein (VLDL)
      (bad) 18, 227, 234
cholinesterase inhibitors 33
chromium ix, 30, 107, 161, 174–80, 238
clonazepam 28
clotting factors 153, 154
co-enzyme Q10 vii, 27, 118–20, 238
  antioxidant properties 124–5, 136–8
  for the circulatory system 29–30, 37,
      63
  inhibitors 65

Coccinia indica 204
cod liver oil 115, 224–5, 227–9
codeine phosphate 27
colds 205–6
coma, hyperglycaemic 7, 38–9
complications of diabetes, long-term 21–40
conjugated linoleic acid vii, 232–4, 238
continuous subcutaneous insulin infusion (CSII) 43
copper 30, 118, 123, 174–5, 181–3
corticosteroids 5, 10, 118
cotton-wool spots 24
Coxsackie B virus 11

danshen 121
death, premature 21, 58, 61, 65, 92, 227
defining diabetes 1–3
dementia 22, 32–3, 213
dextrose tablets 47, 49, 50
diagnosis
    of diabetes 8, 13–16
    of pre-diabetes 19–20
diarrhoea 135
diet vi, 67–91, 235
    as a cause of diabetes 11–12
    eating less 93–4
    traditional approaches 67–70
    types of (for weight loss) 94–104
dieticians 237
dinners 68–9, 69
diuretics 5, 10–11, 39, 60, 122
docosahexaenoic acid (DHA) 77, 78, 224, 227, 229
doctors 92–3, 99, 105, 239
dong quai 121

echinacea 119, 196, 204–7
eczema 231
eicosapentaenoic acid (EPA) 77, 78, 224, 227, 229
embolism 31
epilepsy 171, 232
essential fatty acids (EFAs) 76–80, 83, 120, 223–34, 238
ethnicity 9, 53, 60
evening primrose oil 27, 30, 120, 224, 230–2
exhaustion 7
eye disease 22–5, 28, 111
    antioxidants for 124–5, 128–9, 132–3, 141, 145–6
    B vitamins for 151, 158, 160, 165, 167, 170

herbs for 25, 196, 201–2, 211–12
ezetimibe 65

fats 63, 68–9, 75–83
    see also low-fat diets
    monounsaturated 76, 79–81, 83, 96, 98
    plant sterols and stanols 81, 83
    polyunsaturated 76, 77–80, 83, 96
        see also essential fatty acids
    recommended intake 82–3
    saturated 76–7, 83, 96, 223–4
    trans/hydrogenated 75, 81–3
fatty acids 13, 100
    see also essential fatty acids
    free 17, 46, 53–4
fenugreek 196, 207–8
fibre 68, 72, 88–9, 227
    see also high fibre diets
    insoluble 88–9
    soluble 84, 88–9
fish, oily 35, 77, 78–9, 228
fish oils 29–30, 35, 120, 224–30
fits 50
flavonoids 84, 143
flax seed oil 224, 229
folic acid (folate) 33, 46, 118, 151–2, 154–7, 163, 166–71
food diaries 94
foot problems 27, 34–6, 175, 185–6, 194
free radicals 22, 84, 123, 128
fructosamine tests 48
fruit 31–2, 62, 68, 84–6, 88–9, 102
fungal treatments, topical 119

gamma-linolenic acid (GLA) 77, 224, 230–2
gangrene 22, 35
garlic 29, 30, 34–5, 63, 121, 196, 208–10, 238
gestational diabetes xiii, 5–6
ginkgo biloba 25, 33–5, 37, 119, 121–2, 196, 210–14, 238
ginseng 37, 121, 196, 214–17
glaucoma 24, 25
glitazones 46, 66
glomeruli 22, 26
glucagon 177
glucose
    see also blood sugar (glucose)
    emergency supplies 44, 49, 50, 105
glucose phosphorylation 243
glucose tests (non-fasting/fasting) 14

glucose tolerance
   see also impaired glucose tolerance; oral
      glucose tolerance test
   improving with exercise 242
   improving with herbs 203–4, 207, 209
   improving with micronutrients 139–40,
      176–8, 181, 184–5
glucose tolerance factor (GTF) 161, 176,
   178
GLUT4 243
glutamic acid decarboxylase (GAD) 10
glycaemic index (GI) 64–5, 68–9, 70–3, 75
glycaemic load (GL) 72–3, 86
glycerol 17
glycogen 2–3, 17, 161, 192, 243
glycosylated haemoglobin tests 48
glycosylation 131, 140, 165–6, 210
Gymnema sylvestre 196, 218–19
   extract (GS4) 219

haemorrhage 31
hammer toe 27
heart attack 19, 22, 29–30, 66, 110
   antioxidants for 124, 132–3, 141, 144
   B vitamins for 151, 162, 168
   and diet 78, 80, 84, 88, 103, 110
   essential fatty acids for 227
   and high blood pressure 60, 61, 63
   minerals for 182
heart disease 18, 19–20, 22, 28–31, 53–4,
   64, 110
   antioxidants for 124, 132–3, 137–8,
      140–1, 143–5, 147
   B vitamins for 151, 164, 168–70
   and diet 78–80, 82–5, 87–8, 90, 99
   essential fatty acids for 226–7, 228,
      230
   herbs for 209–10, 222
   and homocysteine levels 152–4
   minerals for 178, 181–2, 185, 193
   symptoms and risks 29–30
   treatments 30–1
   and weight loss 103
heart (cardiac) failure 30, 60, 61, 137–8
herbal medicine viii, ix, 114, 195–222, 239
   directory 198–222
   preparation of herbs 197
   standardised extracts 197–8
   synergy 196–7
   warnings regarding viii–ix
   when to avoid/limit 120–2
heredity 8–9, 17, 64–5, 155–6
high blood pressure 22
   causes 60, 187–8, 190

and diet 79–82, 87, 90–1
   effects 60
   herbs for 209
   measurement 58–9
   micronutrients and 110, 125, 137–8,
      185, 188–9
   in prediabetes 18, 19, 66
   prevalence 58
   symptoms and risks 28
   treatment 28–9, 52, 58–63
high fibre diets 56, 94, 96–7
HLA-DR gene 9
holy basil 196, 220
homocysteine 22, 26, 30, 33–4, 46, 52,
   60, 152–7, 169
   lowering 155–7, 163–4, 166–7, 170–1,
      182
   risks associated with 153
hygiene 36
hypoglycaemia 44, 46–7, 49–50, 88, 93,
   105, 203–4, 239
hypoglycaemic drugs, oral 39, 45–7, 66,
   99, 210–11, 217–19

immune system 205
impaired glucose tolerance (IGT) (border-
   line diabetes) 15, 18, 40, 66, 97
impotence 22, 27, 34, 36–7, 196, 212–13,
   216
infections 7–8, 11, 111, 196, 205–6, 219
inflammation 33, 54, 77, 78
   see also anti-inflammatories
insulin
   actions of 1–3
   in diabetes 3
   and diet 80, 96–7
   essential fatty acids and 233–4
   herbs for 202–3, 207, 210–11, 215,
      218–20
   and high blood pressure 61
   micronutrients and 161, 171, 175, 177,
      185, 191, 193
   and premetabolic syndrome 17–18
   promotion of obesity 17
   and sodium 187, 188
insulin glargine 43
insulin pumps 43
insulin resistance vii, 3, 8
   causes 13, 54, 241
   combating 80, 125, 127, 241, 243
   conditions associated with 39–40
   definition 4–5, 17, 18
insulin sensitivity 56, 125, 127–8, 188,
   243–4

insulin therapy 22–3, 26, 38–9, 42–4, 99, 217
intestinal flora 117
intrinsic factor 166
iodine 174
iron 110, 118, 120, 135, 174, 219
islets of Langerhans 2, 10, 43
isoflavones 85

ketoacidosis, diabetic 7, 37–8, 100–1
ketones 100–1
ketosis 100–1
Ketostix 100
kidney disease 22, 25–6, 28, 60, 126, 135

laxatives 200
legs
    cramping 27, 28
    pain 25–6, 34, 169, 212
    restless 27, 28
leptin 54
life expectancy 21
linoleic acid vii, 77–8, 223–4, 232–4, 238
linolenic acid 77, 223, 224, 229–32
lipase, hormone-sensitive 17
liquid meals 95
liver problems 40, 125, 129, 183
low glycaemic index diets 64–5, 68–9, 75
low-calorie diets 94–5, 103
    see also very low-calorie diets
low-carbohydrate diets 40, 56, 64, 69, 94, 98–104, 249–54
low-fat diets 56, 64–5, 94, 96–7, 103
lunches 68, 69
lutein 25, 124, 127–8
lycopene 128

maggots 36
magnesium 29–30, 35, 63, 107, 110, 115, 118, 120, 174–5, 183–7, 238
magnetic therapy 27
manganese 118, 124, 143, 174
margarine 81, 82
meal-skipping 68
meal-time glucose regulators 46
medical management 41–50, 239
    herbal interactions 120–2
    micronutrient interactions 116–22
    and physical exercise 237
    and weight loss 92–3, 99
meditation 62
metabolic boosters 104–5

metabolic syndrome (pre-diabetes) v, 1–20, 233, 247
    causes 12, 13
    clinical components 17–18
    conditions associated with 24, 39–40
    definition 16–20, 52
    diagnosis 19–20
    and diet 67, 77
    herbs for 218
    and high blood pressure 61
    and homocysteine levels 153
    and insulin resistance 4–5
    lowering your risks of 51, 52–66, 92, 98, 100–1, 103
    and micronutrients 106, 110, 127, 175, 184–5
    multi-treatment approach to 65–6
    and obesity 53–4
    prevalence 16
metformin 40, 45–6, 99, 157, 166
microaneurysms 24
micronutrient supplementation v, vii, 106–22, 237–9
    see also herbal medicine
    additives 112–13, 114
    antioxidants 107–8, 123–49
    benefits of 111
    and diabetic medications 116–22
    essential fatty acids 223–34, 238
    how to take 115–16
    labels 113–14
    lower reference nutrient intake (LRNI) 110
    minerals vi, 106–22, 174–94
    recommended daily amounts (RDAs) 107–8, 113, 116–17
    recommended intake 107–12
    reference nutrient intakes (RNIs) 107, 109–10
    safety issues 111–12
    time-release formulations 113
    units of measurement 108
    vitamin B complex 150–73
    what to look for 112–14
milk, cows' 51
milk thistle 118
minerals
    deficiencies 108–10
    supplementation vi, 106–22, 174–94
mini-stroke 31
molybdenum 174
multiminerals 238
multivitamins 111, 238
mumps 11

muscles 243–4
myelin sheath 22, 27, 77, 125–6
myrtillin 201

nephropathy, diabetic 25–6
nerve problems (diabetic neuropathy)
    22–3, 27–8, 34, 125–6, 151,
    154–6, 158, 164–6, 172–3, 231–2
net carbs 102
nitrosamines 11
non-alcoholic fatty liver disease (NAFLD)
    39–40
non-alcoholic steato-hepatitis (NASH)
    39–40
non-esterified fatty acids (NFAs) 13
non-steroidal anti-inflammatory drugs
    (NSAIDS) 33
nutritional therapists 237–8
nuts 229–30

obesity vi
    anti-obesity drugs for 66, 245–8
    apple-shaped 12–13, 19, 53, 92, 233,
        241
    and conjugated linoleic acid 232–3
    and insulin resistance 17
    measurement 54–6
    and type 2 diabetes 12, 52, 53–8
    and weight loss 95, 97
occupational therapy 32
oils 29–30, 35, 69, 80–1, 120, 224–30
olive oil 80–1
omega-3 essential fatty acids 29–30, 35,
    77–80, 120, 223–30, 224–30
omega-6 essential fatty acids 77–8, 80, 83,
    223–5, 230–2
oral contraceptive pill 118
oral glucose tolerance test (OGTT) 14–15,
    172, 181, 203, 211
orlistat (Xenical) 245–7
osteoporosis 110, 118
overweight vi, 4, 17, 241
    see also obesity

pain
    chest 29–30
    leg 25–6, 34, 169, 212
painkillers 27
panaxans 215
pancreas 1, 3, 41
    beta cells 2, 4, 8–11, 17, 136, 158,
        160, 210–11, 218–20
pancreatic islet cell implants 43
pancreatitis 147–8

paracetamol 27, 118, 119–20
pectin 221–2
phenelzine 217
phenytoin 28
phosphate 118, 174
physical activity 13, 57
physical exercise vi, 56–7, 62, 104–5,
    236–7, 241–4
phytochemicals/phytooestrogens 85
pine bark extracts 124, 145–6, 238
polycystic ovary syndrome 40
polypeptides 73, 202
polyphenols 123, 143
potassium 29, 85, 91, 187–90
pregnancy
    diabetes during ix, 5–6
    essential fatty acids and 229, 234
    herbs to avoid 199–200
    micronutrient and 115, 129–30, 168,
        170–1
    oily fish consumption and 79, 228
    uterine environment during 9, 11
prescription drugs 10–11
prevalence of diabetes vi
prevention of diabetes 51–66
prickly pear 196, 221–2
probiotics 117
prostaglandins 231
protein, dietary 68, 73–5
proteinuria 26
Pycnogenol® 25, 121, 123, 124, 125,
    145–6

quinine sulphate 28

randomised controlled trials 103
Reaven's syndrome see metabolic syndrome
rehydration therapy 38, 39
renin 28, 60
resistin 54
retinopathy, diabetic 22–5, 125, 146, 158,
    165, 167, 201, 211
rhodopsin 127
risk of diabetes, lowering your 51–66
rubella (German measles) 11

St John's wort 121
salt 62–3, 90–1
    see also sodium
scurvy, localised 131
selective serotonin re-uptake inhibitors
    (SSRIs) 119, 121
selenium 30, 85, 123–5, 139, 147–9, 174,
    238

serotonin 121
sibutramine 248
signs/symptoms of diabetes 6–8, 13–14
sildenafil (Viagra) 37
skin, dry 231
skin-prick tests 44
smoking 61–2, 130
snacks 44, 88, 94
sodium 85, 187–91
    see also salt
solid extracts 197
sorbitol formation 131
soya 85
speech therapy 32
spinal cord damage 156, 166
stanols, plant 81, 83
statins 31, 65, 66, 119, 124, 138, 163
sterols, plant 81, 83
stress 62
strokes 18, 19, 22, 28, 31–2, 53, 66
    and diet 78, 80, 83–4, 87, 90–1
    herbs for 213, 222
    and high blood pressure 60, 61, 63
    and homocysteine levels 152, 154
    and micronutrients 110, 132–3, 143,
        145, 168–70, 226–7
    symptoms and risks 31
    treatment 31–2
    types 31
    and weight loss 103
sugar-protein complexes 22
sulphonylureas 45, 46
surgery, vascular 37
syndrome X see metabolic syndrome

tadalafil (Cialis) 37
tea 30, 86–7
    black 63, 86–7, 142–4
    green 63, 86–7, 124, 142–4
    Redbush (rooibosch) 87
    white 63, 86–7, 142–3
tests
    see also oral glucose tolerance test
    diagnostic 14–15
    for glucose levels 47–8, 119, 135
thiazide diuretics 5, 10–11
thirst 7
thrombolytic drugs 32
thrombosis 31
thrush 7, 205, 206
thyroxine 122
tinctures 197
toxins 12
tricyclic antidepressants 119

triglycerides 17–19, 22, 46, 58, 60, 63, 65
    dietary 76
    essential fatty acids and 226, 234
    low-carb diets and 252–4
    lowering with herbs 207–9, 218, 220,
        222
    lowering with micronutrients 139, 162,
        178–9
    measuring levels of 64
    weight loss and 92, 97, 98, 103
twin studies 9
type 1 diabetes (insulin-dependent
        diabetes) v–ix
    and blood sugar control 22–3, 70
    causes 8–12
    in children 44, 128, 160, 165
    complications of 26–8, 37
    definition 3–4
    diagnosis 16
    and diet 70
    herbs for 218
    and hypoglycaemia 49
    medical management 41–4
    micronutrients for 128, 147, 177, 181,
        184, 191–3, 225
    monitoring glucose levels in 41, 44,
        47–8
    and physical exercise 62
    prevention 51–2
    signs/symptoms of 6–7
    and sodium 188
type 2 diabetes (non-insulin dependent/
        maturity onset diabetes) v–ix, 111
    and anti-obesity drugs 247
    antioxidants for 124, 125, 127, 128,
        132, 137–40
    B vitamins for 158–60, 165, 167, 169,
        171–2
    and blood sugar control 23
    causes 8–13, 245
    conditions associated with 24, 26–8,
        30–1, 38–40
    definition 4
    diagnosis 8, 16
    and diet 67, 77, 80
    essential fatty acids and 225–6, 227,
        229, 233
    herbs for 199, 203–4, 208, 210–11,
        213, 215–16, 218–19, 221
    and homocysteine levels 153–4, 155,
        157, 167
    and insulin resistance 4–5, 8, 17
    and low-carb diets 249–50
    lowering your risks of 51, 52–65, 92

and micronutrient deficiencies 110
minerals for 175–7, 179, 181, 184–6,
191–3
monitoring glucose levels in 47–8
and prediabetes 16
signs/symptoms of 7–8
and sodium retention 187
treatment 44–7, 157
and weight loss 92, 98–101, 103, 110,
179, 233

ulcers
of the foot 34–6, 175, 185–6, 194
herbs for 196, 198–9
of the legs 22
urination, excessive (polyuria) 6–7
urine (dip-stick) tests 14, 26
uterine environment 9, 11

vacor 12
vanadium 174, 191–2
vardenafil (Levitra) 37
vascular disease
see also atherosclerosis; blood vessels,
damage to
peripheral 33–4, 151–2, 154, 164, 169,
212
vegetables 31–2, 62, 68, 84–6, 88–9, 102,
150
vegetarians 114, 224, 229–30
very low-calorie diets (VLCDs) 56, 94,
95–6
vision 7, 24, 128–9
see also eye disease
vitamin A 75, 115, 118, 151, 225, 228–9
antioxidant properties 123–5, 127–30
betacarotene 85, 123, 127–30
retinol 127, 129, 130
vitamin B1 (thiamine) 118, 158–9
vitamin B2 (riboflavin) 118, 123, 151,
159–61
vitamin B3 (niacin) 106, 115, 118, 151,
161–3, 180
vitamin B6 (pyridoxine) 118, 151, 154–7,
163–7
vitamin B12 (cyanocobalamin) 46, 118,
151, 154–7, 166–7, 171
vitamin B complex 25–7, 30, 32, 34,
150–73

vitamin C (ascorbic acid) 25, 118, 119–20,
130–4, 194
antioxidant properties 123–5, 130–4
for the circulatory system 30, 31, 32,
34, 37, 132–3
and copper 181
deficiencies 110
recommended intake 108, 134–5
safety issues 135
sources 85, 134
vitamin D 52, 75, 118, 151, 225, 228–9
vitamin E vii–viii, 30, 33, 75, 81, 114,
120, 151, 194, 228
antioxidant properties 123–5, 139–42
deficiencies 110
and essential fatty acids 225
for the eyes 25, 201
recommended intake 142
sources 85, 141–2
vitamin K 117, 120, 151
vitamins
deficiencies 108–10, 150–1
fat-soluble 151
supplementation vii–viii, 106–22,
123–5, 127–35, 139–44,
150–73
see also specific vitamins
water-soluble 151

warfarin 120–2, 214, 217, 228
water consumption 68
weather, cold 11
weight loss 7, 19–20, 26, 56–8, 62,
92–105, 235, 251–2
doctor's advice regarding 92–3, 99, 105
and micronutrients 110, 144, 179,
232–4
physical exercise for 104–5, 241
and types of diet 94–104
weight-to-height ratio charts 55–6
wine 87–8
World Health Organization (WHO) vi,
14, 15, 55

zeaxanthin 128–9
zinc 35, 107, 115, 117–18, 120, 124,
174–5, 183, 192–4